A Personal Guide To
Real-Life Weight Management

GET REAL

DANIEL KOSICH, PhD

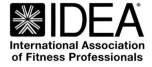

IDEA®
International Association
of Fitness Professionals

Library of Congress Catalog Card Number 95-078637

ISBN: 1-887781-00-5

This information in this book does not constitute medical advice. Before beginning an exercise program, consult a doctor.

Developmental Editor: Mary Monroe

Designer: Paige Hardy & Associates

Copy Editor: Deanne Kells

Printed in the United States of America

Copyright © 1995 by IDEA, Inc.

IDEA, International Association of Fitness Professionals
6190 Cornerstone Court East, Suite 204
San Diego, CA 92121-3773
(619) 535-8979, (800) 999-4332

Acknowledgements

In the more than fifteen years that I have focused attention on the efforts to successfully achieve and maintain a healthy body weight, I have been privileged to share the insights of countless professionals and the frustrations of countless clients who have had the same goal. With far too many names to mention individually, I would like to thank them all for helping me reach my current perspectives on the issue of healthy weight.

More specifically, Barry Molk, MD, Nancy Rodriguez, PhD, RD, James Gavin, PhD, and Ralph La Forge, MS, provided invaluable insights and suggestions in reviewing the concepts presented in this book. They have my deepest thanks and appreciation.

Thanks also to the thousands of IDEA fitness professionals around the world whose commitment and dedication to providing quality programs and building participation in safe and effective fitness programs are key focal points of this book. And to Peter and Kathie Davis, founders of IDEA, the international association of fitness professionals, for their willingness to publish *Get Real*.

Most especially, my profound thanks to Mary Monroe, for her incredible creativity and insightful participation as the developmental editor. Mary's suggestions, input and sensitivity added immeasurably to the final manuscript. Her knowledge regarding body image and self-empowerment issues made these chapters far more meaningful than they would have been had I written them on my own.

This book is dedicated, with love, to my daughters, Anya Danielle and Michelle Ann. Their patience, understanding smiles and encouraging hugs kept me at the keyboard when I'd much rather have been playing with them!

Table of Contents

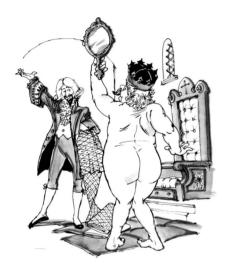

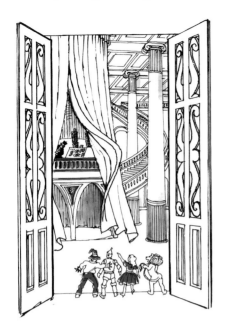

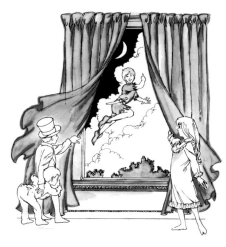

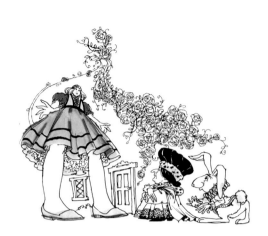

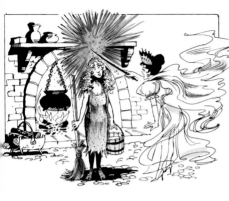

Preface: A Program You Can Live With

This is a book about reality.

In *Get Real*, we're going to look closely at the difference between weight loss fairy tales and real-life solutions. I'll even use a few fairy tales to illustrate key points along the way. I'll also follow the story of one person's lifelong weight struggle, and how she moves from fantasy and disappointment to real-life success. Just as your process of getting healthier should be active and fun, I've tried to make the process of reading this book active and fun!

In addition, I'll provide you with a three-part plan for creating your own healthy weight and healthy living program. It's not an overnight plan, by any means. I'll encourage you to seek out more information in many areas to improve your chances of achieving your goals.

The Reality Factor

What you *will* find in this book is an extremely practical and comprehensive approach to weight management—not just nutrition, not just exercise, not just information on dieting issues or behavior modification or body image, but *all* of those aspects—approached in a realistic and integrated way. More than anything, this book is about the process of learning to be good to yourself through enjoyable healthy habits.

How can you establish a lifestyle that will help you achieve and maintain your own healthy body weight? How can you learn to accept yourself, become more active and eat a nourishing, healthful (and enjoyable!) diet? You'll find out. Don't be in a rush. Take your time. Take it in small steps.

That's how most things happen...in real life.

If there's one thing that's been missing in the endless flood of information on losing weight, it's the "reality factor." But you probably already know that if you've been paying attention to all the wild weight loss ideas around today—and especially if you've ever struggled with weight loss.

Billions of dollars are spent every year for pills, potions and programs which promise to provide, at last, the sure-fire answer to "effective" weight loss. Movie stars, athletes and health experts serve as spokespeople for program X or product Y, citing the incredible benefits it has added to their lives, implying that if you would only try it you'd get the same results. How can you resist?

These pitches are difficult to resist because the fantasy is so tantalizing. Although becoming rich and/or famous are common fantasies, becoming *thin* may be even a more popular modern-day fairy tale. Say a magic word, drink a magic powder, watch a spellbinding diet guru on TV, spin around three times...and you'll be thin enough to wear spandex and star in your own rock video—or at the very least, astonish your friends with the "brand new you" (implying, of course, that the "old you" is easily disposable—and good riddance!).

The *reality* is that for most of us who lose weight, the lost weight—and often, even more—is regained within a relatively short time. Another dose of reality is that this lose/gain cycle potentially increases health risks and, worse, sets the stage for dramatically negative effects on self-image, self-esteem and self-confidence.

In addition, many of us who lose weight (often only to hold on to the coveted goal weight for a few months or so) find another disappointing reality glitch in the fairy tale: Being thin can come conspicuously without fame, fortune, or that part in the rock video! The envy of friends can be oddly unsatisfying, we still don't really look or live like the glamorous people who pitched the products, and most of our old problems are still there. No wonder so many people slip gradually back into their regular habits and end up where they started!

Everywhere we look—magazines, television, newspapers—we see the same message: *The thinner, the better.* "If you want it enough, you can accomplish anything you want to" is the motto we're encouraged to live by.

But it ain't necessarily so.

The fact is that no matter how much I'd like to be the King of Siam, it'll never happen! Research has shown that each of us is so different that for some the quest for the super thin appearance is not only impossible, it's also unhealthy. Genetics plays a key role; we all have to work within our individual traits and capabilities. How our bodies respond to weight loss programs, our personal preferences for various foods and nutrients, and a host of other physiological and psychological factors, all interrelated (and many of which science has not even begun to understand fully), make up our own unique weight management profile. With such an intricate interplay of factors, you can understand all the more why gimmicks and tricks can't work!

Finding the Middle Ground

Are we doomed to be stuck forever somewhere between fat and fantasy?

The answer is, No!

That's what *Get Real* is about. Between the extreme fads (and futility) of fairy tale thinness and the risky extreme of sedentary living and unhealthy weight, *there is a middle ground.* This middle ground is what I mean by real-life weight management—a way of living that is sensible, healthy and attainable for *real people*, with real appetites and attitudes, real families and jobs, real schedules and real budgets.

Real-life weight management may be a little disappointing for people who are still looking for a fairy godmother or a magic lamp to whisk away fat. But the beauty of real-life weight management is that it brings *real-life magic*—like feeling better and looking better, enjoying new activities and satisfying new accomplishments, liking who you are more, making healthy activity and food choices out of self-respect and enjoyment rather than guilt, looking forward to a longer, healthier, happier life—and, yes, even reasonable, *lasting* weight loss.

How can you resist?

In real life, weight is not an isolated factor that can be "controlled" without regard for the whole person. This is another good reason why simple solutions for quick, easy weight loss have proven so useless. Your interests, attitudes, feelings, background, biology, lifestyle and more all play a part.

We do know that weight is just one aspect of overall health.

And your best opportunity to achieve and maintain a healthy weight is to practice overall healthy living. The real-life weight management process that I will outline in *Get Real* has three essential components:

- self-empowerment (including self-acceptance)

- active living

- sensible eating.

Most diets and plans in the past have focused almost exclusively on various food solutions—what to eat and what not to and how much and when and where and on and on. Real-life weight management is about much more than just food, for two main reasons:

- Being as active as possible is an important key. A sensible diet (but not a highly restrictive one) is important as part of an active lifestyle.

- It's hard to get motivated to adopt healthy living habits if you don't feel good about yourself—and don't empower yourself to take action (and maintain it).

The Reality of Eating Disorders

It is extremely important to recognize that eating disorders are also a very real aspect of the health and weight risk picture. Anorexia and bulimia are perplexing, poorly understood behaviors. Binge eating and the various forms of overeating behavior which occur across the weight spectrum are even less understood. It is encouraging that researchers are exploring these areas today, and that organizations such as the National Association of Anorexia Nervosa and Associated Disorders are making strides in the treatment of these difficult problems.

If you suspect that an eating disorder may play a part in your weight loss struggles or patterns, I urge you to seek help and information. There are many compassionate and knowledgeable professionals who can help you understand and move beyond the pain of eating-disordered behavior.

It is beyond the scope of this book to address eating disorders, which require treatment by qualified specialists. However, successful eating disorder treatment often can set the stage for implementing the general healthy weight and healthy living guidelines presented in *Get Real*.

Section I. Exposing the Naked Truth
(Or, Why the Emperor Who Diets Has No Clothes)

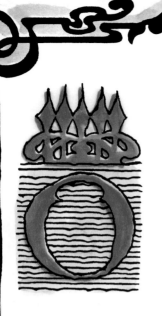

nce upon a time, a great emperor decided he wanted the most fabulous outfit he could find for a really big parade that was coming up. He assembled all the best tailors in the royal town to come up with designs for him—Sir Calvin Kind, The Dutchess Glorious Vandersilk, Perry Trellis, even Georgio Ourmoney.

All of the tailors showed him very lavish, Hollywood-type duds, but the emperor was unimpressed—that is, until the last tailor appeared. He was a relative unknown, but what a proposal! He danced and twitched and stitched in thin air as he unclothed the emperor and went through the motions of dressing him in invisible (but allegedly exquisite!) finery.

"Isn't that the most incredible look you've ever seen!" cried the tailor. "This is going to do wonders for your image, sir, and the best thing about it is that only the most hip, intelligent, sophisticated people can see this absolutely revolutionary design!"

Now, the emperor honestly only saw his usual naked self in the mirror, but he really wanted the townspeople to be impressed and he didn't want to let on that he might not be all that hip and sophisticated, so he said nothing.

The rest is history. The emperor went down in the books as an unfortunate flasher, all because he sold out his honest convictions for a great-sounding bill-of-goods—the promise of a fabulous new image.

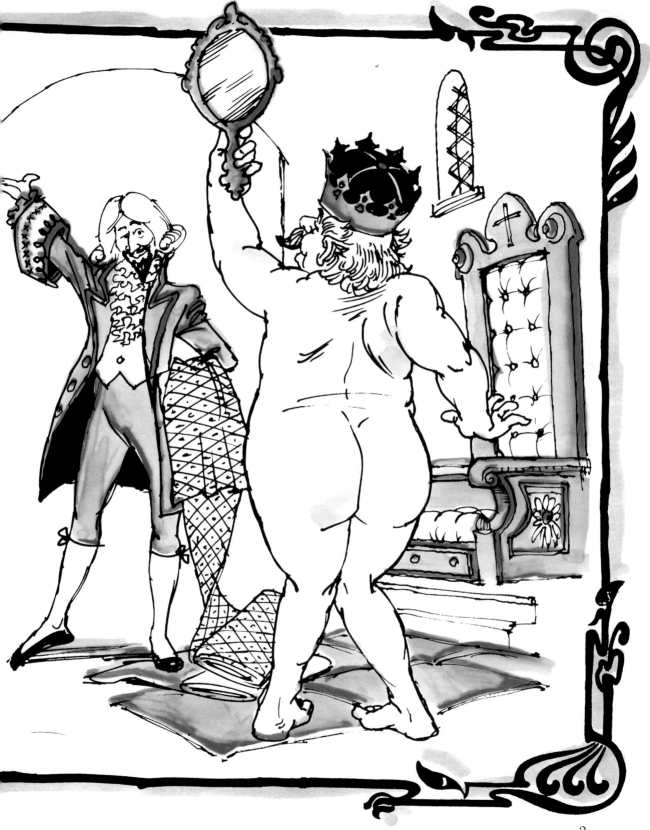

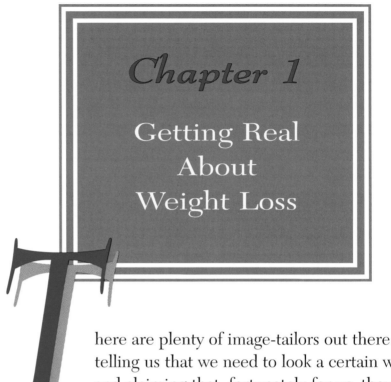

Chapter 1

Getting Real About Weight Loss

There are plenty of image-tailors out there telling us that we need to look a certain way and claiming that, fortunately for us, they've got the magic answer to make it happen. Their promises are so irresistible that it's often hard to listen to the little, down-to-earth, honest voice inside that's saying, *"Wake up! There are no magic formulas for weight loss. And besides, why does everyone have to look the way these people want us to?"*

It sounds so logical, but any of you who've been there know that the weight loss struggle can get the best of you—literally. How many people have given month after dieting month— and ultimately some or most of the best years of their lives— to doing battle with their weight? This is one of those better-kept secrets that is only surfacing today as more brave people talk about what it's like to suffer with a weight problem (real or imaginary, and we have plenty of both).

The more popular thinking has generally been that anybody can lose weight with "a little willpower." People with weight problems have been labeled lazy or greedy or just lacking in moral character. Through exposure to TV and billboards, we have gotten used to seeing thin, joyful people dancing out of their big-size clothes, saying, "I did it, and it was easy, with _____!" Since most of the people that we ever see in any media are conspicuously thin, it isn't surprising that we're beginning to believe that thin is normal.

But fortunately that's changing, little by little, as we begin to uncover the truth about weight issues. At last, we are beginning to understand two crucial factors that make an enormous difference in how we approach weight management:

- There is no one "normal" body size, no matter what we see on the TV or movie screen.
- There's nothing easy about struggling with a weight problem.

Don't get me wrong—I am going to talk about effective weight loss strategies in this book, but first I want to establish a real-life perspective on this whole area of weight loss. As I said, this factor has been sorely lacking in most approaches.

How Maggie Tried…and Why Maggie Is Tired of Trying

"I'm such a failure."

Those are Maggie's silent words as she stares at herself in the bathroom mirror. Tomorrow is her 38th birthday. Maggie looks at the listless, tired woman in the mirror—and all she feels is shame.

The talk inside her head begins.

"I've tried everything I can think of and I'm still fat. Maybe I'll get myself that Fat-Buster spring I saw on TV last night as a birthday present to myself. What'd he say? 'Guaranteed to shrink four inches off your waist in a month!' Or maybe that video program with that gorgeous instructor who said I could look just like her in only 20 minutes a day, three times a week."

Wryly, Maggie thinks to herself, "I wonder if she works out for only 20 minutes, three times a week?"

Thinking back, it feels to Maggie like she's been trying to lose weight her whole life. She still remembers the time in fourth grade when those boys called her "Fatty" and made fun of her while she was eating her bologna sandwich and coconut cupcake.

Maggie felt ashamed and hurt and angry. Why was there something wrong with her? She became more and more self-conscious as she grew older, always wondering if people were finding something wrong with how she looked.

In high school, several teachers discovered Maggie's talent for drawing and encouraged her to pursue her art. Maggie began to dream about becoming a graphic designer. She worked hard on developing her skills, but she worked even harder at losing weight. She skipped school lunches and even got excited when one of her friends told her all she had to do to lose weight was make herself throw up after she ate.

Maggie wanted to go to the high school prom so much. But who'd ask her if she didn't lose some weight? She was still bigger than most of her friends.

"Okay," she decided, "I'll just cut way back on eating. No breakfast and just a soda for lunch."

Trouble was, by the time she got home in the evening she was so hungry that she'd eat a whole bag of cookies or chips. There were times when she would eat hardly anything for days—and it seemed to work, too! She'd lose weight after a couple of weeks or months. In fact, she even squeezed into a size 8 prom dress.

But it was hard to enjoy the prom; all night she kept comparing herself to the other girls, who all seemed to be size 4 or 6. She kept wondering if her date thought she was still too big. After the prom she couldn't keep the starvation regimen up, and as usual, all the weight slipped back on before she knew it.

When Maggie was in college, one of her friends told her the real answer to losing weight was to exercise. "You've got to burn more calories than you eat."

Dutifully Maggie went to the gym with the commitment of an athlete and started losing weight! But she felt terrible—irritable, no energy—and her grades started dropping. After a couple of months she just couldn't do it anymore, so she stopped. The weight started coming back on, fast.

Everywhere Maggie looked, the messages were clear:

Lose Weight, Be More Sexy

Lose Weight, Be Happier

Lose Weight, Be Healthier

Lose Weight, Have More Friends

Lose Weight, Have More Fun

TV commercials, clothing catalogs, radio advertisements, magazine ads, billboards, it was everywhere! Models spread the message: "Whatever you do, don't get fat." It didn't matter what the product was—clothes, cigarettes, alcoholic beverages, vacations, cars...it was a constant topic of conversation.

In her last year of college, Maggie met Jim. It was at just about the same time that she heard about the latest weight loss powder. "Maybe I've finally found the answer! I really like him. I'll use this program for a couple of months until I lose 15 pounds. Then I can go back to eating regular. Forget the exercise, it was too much work."

Sure enough, two months later Maggie had lost the 15 pounds she'd wanted to. Jim told her how proud of her he was. "You're lookin' great," all her friends were saying.

"At last," she thought, "I've done it. I'm so tired of this weight loss powder. It's so boring. It's going to be great to eat real food again." By then she and Jim were engaged to be married. She loved being with Jim, and one thing she especially, secretly loved was that he didn't seem to think there was anything wrong with how she looked. Maggie thought that made Jim very unique indeed.

Within six months of going back to her regular habits Maggie had regained not just the 15 pounds she had lost, but 5 pounds more. And she hated herself for it. "What's wrong with me? It felt so good to wear that size 8. Now look at me. I can't believe how weak-willed I am."

At the wedding, when everyone told her how beautiful she looked, all Maggie could think was, "Yeah, right, but nowhere near as good as I did six months ago."

Maggie gained another 5 pounds in the first six months after the wedding. She started to believe she felt subtle pressure from Jim to lose some weight. It seemed like he wasn't quite as affectionate. Her friends weren't telling her how good she looked anymore. She couldn't get into the clothes she was so excited about six months ago. Then she found out she was pregnant.

Maggie's doctor made it clear that now was not the time to try to lose weight. Her self-esteem hit an all-time low, and she just couldn't keep from eating a lot. She was very excited about the baby, but she felt so big that she didn't even want to look in the mirror. She couldn't wait to lose weight after she had the baby. It was almost all she could think about.

Six months after the baby was born, Maggie heard about a program where she could go once a week to be weighed. Then she could buy all of her meals for a week, prepackaged. She wouldn't have to cook anything— except for Jim, that is.

"Maybe this is the answer," she thought. "I'll try it. They even have contests to win free packaged meals for the one who loses the most weight each week. We're going on vacation in a month and I want to lose at least

20 pounds before we leave. Five pounds a week. They tell me that if I stick with it I could actually lose 30 pounds in 30 days. Yes! Then I can lose the rest after we get back." Once again, she started losing weight quickly. "Maybe I can get Jim to try this, too—he could stand to lose a few pounds."

Jim's response was simple: No way! So, Maggie found herself preparing most of the meals for her husband, while eating the prepackaged meals for herself. Talk about self-control. Halfway through the month she was getting pretty tired of her meals, and the expense.

"Maybe I'll just eat a little bit of what I make for Jim. No, I won't. I can do this. I've got a goal and I'm going to make it." So, she stayed with her diet program and lost 25 pounds before they went on vacation. She was quite proud of herself. "I made it," she thought.

Trouble struck. Without the prepackaged meals and with the excitement of vacation, she and Jim had a great time exploring the variety of restaurants in the area. It was sure nice to be eating a wide variety of tasty meals again!

Back from two weeks of vacation, she'd regained 5 pounds of the 25 she had lost. "No problem, I'll just go back on my diet program," Maggie thought. But it wasn't much fun. She often thought about how much better it would be just to eat what she was making for her husband.

With great determination, Maggie stayed with the diet program for two months, losing 35 pounds. But then it just got to be too much trouble. It was boring, she was tired of having to go every week, and it was pretty expensive.

Maggie gave up and went back to her old habits. She became depressed and found herself eating to help her be less depressed. Six months later she'd regained all of her weight and felt worse about herself than ever. Then came her second baby.

Over the next 15 years Maggie tried many more ways to lose weight—health clubs, diet pills, the latest device to burn the fat on her tummy and inner thighs. She spent lots of money, made herself not eat things she liked, made herself eat things she didn't like, and felt more and more like it was becoming harder and harder to lose weight and easier and easier to gain it. After the latest attempt—two weeks at a spa where they fed her almost nothing and had her climbing hills and riding bikes until she was exhausted—she'd lost 12 pounds in 14 days. But the weight was back on in three months.

So, now, here she was, in front of her mirror on the day before her 38th birthday, wondering if she should even try to lose weight before her 20-year high school reunion coming up in six months. And wondering what had happened to the last 20 years.

Her life was so stressful with the kids and her job at the bank. She and Jim hardly had time to see each other—it was hard to even know how she felt about him anymore. Somehow, she'd forgotten about a lot of her dreams and plans—like being an artist. What had happened to them? She'd just been so busy, but doing what?

Suddenly it hit her. Maggie realized, with shock and dismay, exactly what had kept her busy for the last 30 years: trying to lose weight.

Maggie stared at herself and knew she was losing hope.

Maybe she'd even already lost hope.

Do You Know Someone Like Maggie?

Does Maggie's story—all the gaining and losing and gaining—make you tired just to think about? The fact is, Maggie's story makes *Maggie* tired. And if you've been through this cycle yourself, you know the feeling.

How does it happen that a bright, talented woman loses precious decades of her life to anguish over *weight*? Though many stories are less dramatic than Maggie's (and a lot of others involve more severe consequences), the truth is that we have not really faced up to the serious impact that preoccupation with weight control and the practice of ineffective methods has had on our lives.

There are no statistics on how many families have been affected, but it may be more accurate to ask if there are many families that have not been affected in some way or another by a member's struggle with weight.

Half of the women and a third of the men in the United States are on a diet on any given day...People who feel that they need to weigh what they did in high school...Others who feel that the only way they'll ever be happy with themselves and life in general is if they can lose weight...People who feel that if they just have enough willpower they can at last lose the weight they want to.

Like Maggie, many have given up hope. Or they're hoping against hope that the latest quick fix weight loss approach will work. (And our fixation with thinness is not just an adult problem. Eating disorders have become nearly an epidemic problem in teenage girls.)

The paradox is that even with so much time, energy and money spent on losing weight, the research tells us that as a society, *both kids and adults are getting heavier than ever*.

Yes, indeed, we've created a huge problem, both in our perceptions and in our behaviors. Immense amounts of effort and emotion have been expended, with little result. The weight loss struggle continues for many, many people like Maggie, building its own unhealthy momentum of desperation, discontent and problematic living habits.

Where did we go wrong?

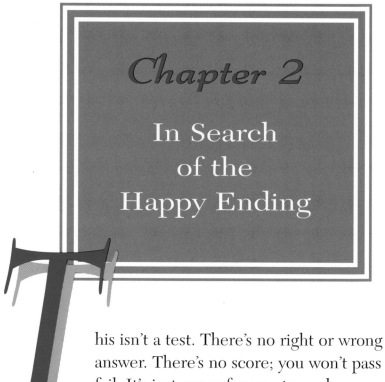

Chapter 2

In Search of the Happy Ending

This isn't a test. There's no right or wrong answer. There's no score; you won't pass or fail. It's just a way for you to explore some of your thoughts and feelings regarding your weight and the way you look at yourself. Write them down in this book, like a journal. Don't just think about them. Writing will take a little longer, but it'll also make you think about your ideas a little more. You will also be able to refer back to what you've written in the *Question Check-Back* sections that occur throughout the book. Above all, you'll be able to watch your progress as your perspectives change.

If you're reading right past this without any intention of writing anything down, that's fine. Just keep in mind that although getting ideas from this book doesn't depend on your participation, getting *results* does. And remember that regardless of how much of this book you implement right now, you can always do more later, when you're ready. The whole point is to take one step at a time—and take them at *your* pace.

Ten Questions to Start Getting Real

As you write down your responses to these 10 questions, try to think about how much your feelings are influenced by what you've seen and heard in magazines, on television, in advertising, and from friends, family and so forth. Remember, your thoughts aren't right or wrong, they're just the way you feel right now. Write as little or as much as you feel like writing—but try to write something.

1. What do you think about your body weight? How often do you think about your weight?

_____

_____

_____

_____

2. How many times in the last five years have you tried to lose weight? How long did you keep it off?

_____

_____

_____

3. How have you tried to lose weight? If you've tried more than once, mention all the ways you've tried.

_____

_____

_____

_____

4. If you lost weight, then gained it back, why do you think that happened?

_____

_____

_____

5. Why do (did) you want to lose weight?

_____
_____
_____
_____

6. When you look at yourself in front of a mirror without your clothes on, what do you see? If you lost weight how would your life change?

_____
_____
_____
_____

7. When you see others successfully lose weight, and you can't, what do you feel?

_____
_____
_____
_____

8. Do you agree with this statement: "The reason you can't successfully lose weight is that you don't have enough willpower to stay with your weight loss program"?

_____
_____
_____
_____

9. How many pounds do you think you need to lose to feel successful about your weight management program?

_____
_____
_____

10. What do you think when you see or hear an advertisement for the latest weight loss program or product?

_____
_____
_____

The reason these questions are important for you to answer is so that you can begin to be more aware of your own feelings and attitudes. It is easy to get caught up in all the messages we see and hear about weight, without realizing what our *own* messages are. Often, we find that we have started to tell ourselves exactly the things we have seen and heard around us—whether or not we really want to believe these messages, much less base our behavior on them.

As you read this book you will have the opportunity to compare your thoughts and feelings with the real-life weight management ideas I present here. You might want to keep some of your ideas, discard some, and, I hope, add some new ones as you start your own journey to "get real" about your weight and your lifestyle.

Many people's answers to questions like these reflect how most weight management programs have created more problems than helpful, realistic, individual solutions. They have perpetuated unrealistic expectations and presented few realistic solutions.

In the 15 years that I've worked with universities and in the fitness industry, I've known hundreds of people who wanted to lose weight. Some needed to; others didn't, but thought they did. And some needed to gain weight! Like many in the field, it always disturbed me that so few of my clients were able to achieve long-term, lifetime success.

In my own experience with many clients trying to lose weight, I have had to "get real" about my ideas and attitudes. There once was a time when I thought that clients weren't getting long-term success simply because they weren't trying hard enough. I explained the lack of success with ideas like, "they aren't staying with the program," "they aren't accurately recording their eating and exercise habits," or any of a number of other objective, scientific reasons that I hoped could explain the situations.

Today I think I was missing some of the most important pieces—namely, the powerful messages, myths and misconceptions that have done so much damage to our weight management efforts, and ultimately, to our overall health. I like to think that the process of "getting real" starts with letting go of three wishes.

Because we all wanted to believe in the easy happy ending, where we could look like what we wanted, eat what we wanted, be wonderfully healthy, and live happily ever after, we were eager to hope that our wildest weight wishes would be granted.

There are three wishes in particular that have done more damage than any doughnut ever could. Let's look at them one at a time.

WISH NO. 1: We Wanted To Believe in Magic

Isn't human nature interesting? We wanted to believe, like the emperor, in a magic solution—no matter how far-fetched! No matter how many times we hear the experts tell us that there's no magic to a certain process, we still want to believe that there is. Weight management is certainly no exception. If I told you a pill had just been formulated that would instantly help you lose weight, would you be writing down its name—even before you found out about the side effects?

By the way, there are medications currently available which purport to help some people get to or maintain a healthier weight. However, they don't offer a "magic" answer, by any means. To be considered are all the very real aspects that always accompany medication, especially lifelong medication, including potential side effects, individual responses and variations, and expense, to name a few.

I've had clients who have tried a multitude of "secret formulas." Magic powders in cans. Magic pills to burn fat while you sleep. Magic belts to burn fat while you sit. Magic weeks at a spa where you'll become a new person, losing pounds and pounds in the process.

But, sadly, while many of these approaches have led to significant weight loss for a short period, the vast majority of clients have regained the weight within a couple of years.

Disappointment, anger, lowered self-esteem, feelings of failure, despair, and ultimately, obsession, have led many to be even more willing to try the next secret formula.

The truth is that we have to let go of the hope for a magic solution. Each of us has to do it for ourselves. The secret is that there is no secret.

The truth is that we're quite a long way from having many answers at all to the mysteries of weight management— much less magic ones. You're not the only one who has been frustrated in your search for solutions. There's a lot that *nobody* knows about weight management.

Question Check-Back

When you answered questions 2, 3, 4, 6, 8 and 10, were any of your responses based on a hope for some new discovery or secret formula which will get you to your goal?

WISH NO. 2: ## We Wanted a One-Size-Fits-All Answer

Think for a moment. How many aspects of real life are the same for everybody? How much control do we have over the color of our eyes? The color of our skin? Whether (like me!) we'll still have our hair when we're 45? How tall we'll grow? How big our feet and hands are?

Of course, we don't have control over any of these things. Yet, as a society, we've created the impression that all of us need to be at a body weight where we look like the models, both women and men, who endlessly appear before us in advertising and entertainment.

A client of mine, Ruth, said to me one day, "A friend of mine and I decided to give it a try. What did we have to lose? So, we did everything just the way we were told. We ate just the packages of food we were given, did our 30 minute walk 3 days a week, and went to the weekly meetings. But after 6 weeks, she'd lost 15 pounds and I'd only lost 6 pounds. It's so unfair. What did I do wrong?"

Ruth is right, it's not always fair. Nobody said it was going to be fair. The truth is that we're all very different. And there are some things, like body weight, which are influenced by factors which we can't control. Our genetics, for example.

While scientists have suspected it for a long time, it's only been recently that several genetic factors have been identified which leave no doubt that body weight is definitely influenced by genetic makeup. Three of the most important are:

- the number of fat cells on your body
- your resting metabolic rate
- the set point theory

Your Number of Fat Cells

The number of fat cells you have on your body has a strong influence on your body weight. John Foreyt, PhD, and G. Ken Goodrick, PhD, tell us in *Living Without Dieting* that by the time you reach adulthood, you have around 30 billion fat cells. Fat cells are a very important part of your body, primarily as a storage tank for energy, just like the gas tank in your car. But some people might have only 25 billion while others might have 35 billion.

A difference of 10 billion fat cells is a lot! Fat cells can get bigger and smaller, but they don't ever go away. So, if Ruth has 10 billion more fat cells than her friend, that could be at least part of the reason why they responded so differently to the same program.

Another important point about fat cells: if you gain a lot of extra weight, like 40 to 50 pounds or more above your healthy weight, you can make billions of new fat cells, which also won't ever go away. This undoubtedly helps explain why some people have an impossible time reaching the weight loss goal calculated strictly on calories-in/calories-out arithmetic or height/weight chart estimates.

Your Metabolism

The word **metabolism** simply refers to all of the processes your body goes through every day: building and repairing cells, producing energy to keep you breathing, keeping your heart pumping, your brain working, your muscles taking you up and down stairs, and all the rest. *Resting metabolic rate* is the number of calories burned just in the essential processes—heart beating, breathing, brain "thinking," etc.

Guess what? By genetic makeup some people have a higher resting metabolic rate than others. So, they burn more calories every day—and it doesn't have anything to do with exercise. Since resting metabolic rate accounts for as much as 70% of daily calories burned in a sedentary person, this certainly helps us understand why some people can eat more than others and not gain weight, even though they're less active.

There's also some suspicion that the body chemistry changes produced by "yo-yo" dieting—lose weight, gain weight, lose weight, gain weight—might have long-term effects on a person's tendency to put on body fat more easily, and to have a more difficult time losing fat. (While the issue of yo-yo dieting's impact on metabolic rate remains controversial, we do know for certain that it can have a devastating impact on self-confidence and motivation for many people.)

Set Point Theory

Question Check-Back

How did you answer questions 1, 2, 4, 5, 6, 7, 8 and 10? Were any of your answers influenced by the reality that one person's ideal weight is another person's impossible (and unnecessary) dream?

Growing evidence suggests that a very important control center in the brain, called the hypothalamus, plays a crucial role in regulating body fat and body weight. Some liken it to the thermostat in your home. If the house gets too cold, the thermostat turns on the furnace to bring up the heat. If the house gets too hot, the thermostat shuts off the furnace to cool things down.

The set point theory may work in a similar fashion. If you eat too many calories, the set point kicks up your metabolism to maintain your body fat level. If you eat too few calories, the set point slows down your metabolism to conserve energy in an attempt to maintain your weight.

Strong support for the set point theory comes from the typical response of returning to previous weight when going off low-calorie diets. This is compelling evidence that something in our body is fighting to maintain a genetically predetermined weight.

20

All this genetic stuff certainly doesn't mean that you're destined to be obese, or that there'll never be a way for you to lose weight if you need to. What it does mean is that your progress through a sensible, real-life weight management program will be unique. And it also means that your ultimate healthy weight might be higher than what you have imagined.

WISH NO. 3: We Thought the Answer Was All-or-Nothing

When a client, Bill, and I were talking about his previous attempts to lose weight, it struck me that his impressions are probably shared by a lot of people.

"I gave it my best," he said. "Exercised five days a week, 10-15 minutes a day, as hard as I could. I was exhausted, even in such a short time. I gave up desserts and red meat, ate salad for lunch, and asked for popcorn without butter at the movies."

I asked him, "Did you look forward to your exercise program? How about eating, were meals something you looked forward to?"

"Heck, no! I was still sore from exercising after about a month, and I couldn't wait for a hamburger and fries. So, pretty soon I started skipping exercise days and grabbing foods I knew I shouldn't eat. Now, here I am. I've regained not just the 10 pounds I lost, but 15. And I'm certainly not excited about starting that program again."

Sound at all familiar?

For many of us, the all-or-nothing approach has been what we thought we had to do. Exercise meant do-or-die, supported by the no pain, no gain theory. If you didn't feel like a truck had run over you by the end of your workout, then you hadn't worked out hard enough! Healthy eating meant tofu, eggplant, rice cakes and carrots forever.

Elaborate, carefully constructed daily and weekly plans have been conceived for exercise and nutrition habits that only about seven people on the entire planet will ever be able to stick to! After a while, for most of us, the nutrition plan becomes so boring or time consuming that it just doesn't work as part of real life. And Bill wondered why he ended up on his couch dreaming of cookies, hamburgers and candy bars!

There's a good reason why we came up with this wish. Extremes often seem easier than finding the moderate way. Black and white can seem much more comforting than that grey area. "Yes" and "No" instructions are direct and easy to follow, but "Maybe" requires ongoing use of judgment. Eating one salad and a chicken breast every day for lunch is a plan that leaves no room for confusion or error. Unfortunately, human beings do not naturally function very well in most all-or-nothing scenarios.

Question Check-Back

How did you answer questions 3, 4, 7, 8 and 9? Any all-or-nothing thinking in your responses?

It is precisely because of the need for ongoing use of judgment that a person in search of effective weight management must develop the ability to make good choices through self-awareness, self-acceptance and ultimately self-empowerment. And that is why I will begin the *Get Real* approach by discussing these essential but often overlooked areas.

Losing Weight IS Possible

We see the infomercial stars telling us:

"They're wrong and I'm right."

"You've tried their way, and it didn't work, right? Try mine and I guarantee it'll work!"

"This fantastic new machine is *the best* and *only* way to effectively lose weight."

Question Check-Back

Look again at question 5. Hopefully, your response emphasizes being more healthy. Yes, appearance is important—but not at the expense of self-confidence and enjoyable living. Losing weight is possible for almost anyone who really needs to. It just may not be in the way or amount you thought.

The fact that people buy into these words is sad. That business is booming for companies whose advertising claims are unrealistic and untrue is disturbing. And that many of us buy these products again and again is discouraging. But there are others who are giving up entirely. The alarming statistics on eating disorders and our increasingly schizophrenic eating habits that bounce from no-fat to loaded-with-fat, from miniscule portions to giant portions, indicate that we're moving toward two ways of thinking: a life-consuming obsession with food, weight and fitness, and a "Who-cares-I-give-up-it's-not-worth-the-trouble" attitude.

That's sad. Because neither extreme is healthy.

You *don't* have to give up and you *don't* have to become obsessed with weight control. As we're letting go of the ideas that didn't work, we're finding some things that do. They may not be as glamorous as the old "magic one-size-fits-all-do-or-die" thinking. But real-life weight management has one big advantage—you can live with it.

Real people, like you and me, with families, jobs and time constraints, can live with it. And that's what I want to tell you about from here on out.

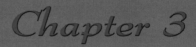

How Real-Life Magic Works

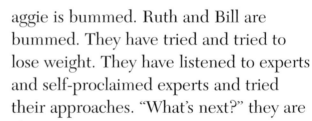aggie is bummed. Ruth and Bill are bummed. They have tried and tried to lose weight. They have listened to experts and self-proclaimed experts and tried their approaches. "What's next?" they are thinking—and maybe you are, too. Let's go back to Maggie's story, and listen as she is introduced to real-life weight management.

Maggie's Challenge

"I really do want to lose weight before my 20-year high school reunion," Maggie thought to herself. *"After having had weight problems all through school, it'd be great to show up looking fit and trim. That would sure surprise everyone! But I don't want to just lose the weight and then put it right back on again...."*

That's when I met Maggie, and it didn't take long for me to sense the challenge in her demeanor. She was polite enough as we introduced ourselves and she told me her long history of dieting attempts and ultimate failures, but I could also hear some of the thoughts she wasn't saying:

"Yeah, right, so, what is it that you're going to be able to offer that I haven't already tried? And I know all that stuff about the health risks of obesity—heart disease, diabetes, high blood pressure, gall bladder problems, stress and strain on my hips, knees and ankles. I don't want another lecture about why it's important for me to lose some weight. I know it is, otherwise I wouldn't be here."

What Maggie dared to ask me aloud was, "What's the story on this real-life weight management thing?"

"The story," I told her, "is that we're finally beginning to understand that all of the control-crazy approaches to weight management simply don't work for most people. Contrary to popular misconception, people who have tried time and again to lose weight probably have more self-control than anyone! Those who haven't ever gone through six weeks of controlled dieting ought to try it some time if they want an experience in self-control!"

Maggie nodded in agreement. She seemed surprised that I understood the rigorous demands of lifelong dieting. She clearly was not used to receiving much acknowledgment for the monumental efforts she'd made.

I continued. "But we know from research data that the vast majority of the highly disciplined people who lose weight regain it when they return to a more realistic lifestyle. So, what seems to be important is to try to put weight management into the same perspective as most other things we do: take it a day at a time, be sensible, but don't try to force a regimen which is so strict that you know from the outset that you couldn't live this way for the rest of your life." I concluded, "The reality is that you *have* to live with it for the rest of your life."

"Sounds like a life sentence," Maggie said cynically. (I was starting to like her down-to-earth attitude!)

I answered, carefully: "Maggie, I could try to tell you that we can put you on a program for six weeks or three months or a year and a half, and when it's over, the weight would be gone forever and you could go back to your old way of living," I said. "But we both know that wouldn't be honest. The bottom line for any behavior change is just that—change. There's that old saying, 'If you always do what you've always done, you'll always get what you've always gotten.'

"I wouldn't be doing my job if I didn't tell you that weight loss is going to mean making some permanent changes. The key to remember is that together we can figure out a way to make these changes *reasonable* and *practical* for you. We're not going to create a program that would necessarily work for a movie star, or for your neighbor, or for your mother. We're going to design it specifically for *you*."

"If I lose the weight—that's what matters," Maggie said bluntly.

"As a matter of fact, what you're probably going to learn in this process is that losing weight *isn't* all that matters. Being healthy and full of energy, learning to know yourself better and like yourself, learning to be compassionate with yourself, being able to respond to stress in a productive way, being able to align your lifestyle with your personal values—all of these go hand in hand with healthy living. Don't forget that we aren't just planning to get you to a magic goal weight and that will be the end of it! We're going to start a new way of living that has to be rewarding enough for you to want to stick with it even when the extra pounds are gone and your motivation to lose this weight isn't there anymore.

"As far as losing the weight, we're going to try to design an approach which will enable you to reach a reasonable goal—a goal based on your own unique situation, in terms of both your physiology and your lifestyle. In all honesty, Maggie, I'm not going to tell you what you'll ultimately be able to weigh. Because I don't know! But I do know that with patience and persistence you'll be able to lose some weight."

What I most wanted Maggie to understand was that she didn't have to lose hope—it *is* possible to achieve a healthy weight. Magic and happy endings aren't just for fairy tales! But she would have to understand that real-life magic doesn't usually happen the way it does in books and movies. And sometimes the happy ending is a different happy ending than the one we imagined!

1, 2, 3, Presto…The Real Life Program

As I discussed earlier, to begin real-life weight management, we first need to let go of the belief in a "single" solution. The answer does not lie in food alone, exercise alone, emotional health, spiritual health or any other single-minded approach. Instead, we need to approach weight management as something that works much the way we know from modern physics and chemistry that everything else in the world works: as a dynamic, ongoing interaction of *many* factors.

The primary factors in real-life weight management can be summarized with three key areas: self-empowerment, activity habits and eating habits.

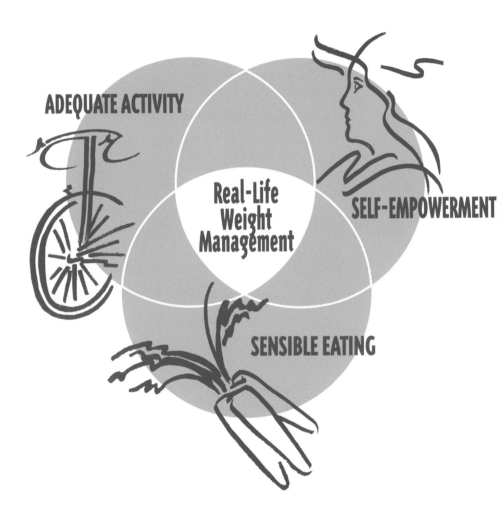

ADEQUATE ACTIVITY

SELF-EMPOWERMENT

Real-Life
Weight
Management

SENSIBLE EATING

Before we go any further, let's clarify one thing: we will not be spending the rest of this book talking about how you can achieve a perfect balance in each of these three areas for the rest of your life. Life just doesn't work that way. What we will be talking about is how you can *gradually* create a *better* balance for yourself in these areas—not every day, but most days. The factors are not separate. Sometimes we rush from one to another, viewing them as separate and independent factors. But they're not.

Like most things in life, each of these areas is constantly changing for all of us, bringing unexpected—and sometimes very difficult—challenges. But these challenges don't have to spell disaster for our healthy living plan. Because what matters isn't what we do for a short period, like six weeks or six months. What matters is what we do most of the time, on a regular, consistent basis, over the course of a lifetime.

The 80/20 Answer

I explained to Maggie that each of the three real-life weight management factors can be thought of as a three-dimensional sphere, constantly interacting with the other two. "It's this interaction which ultimately impacts body weight," I explained.

"What do you mean, interaction?" she asked.

"Well, all three of the spheres are constantly changing. On some days you feel better about yourself than on other days. You might get sick and be unable to exercise for a week. At a special dinner you might eat a T-bone steak, a baked potato with butter and sour cream, and a hot fudge sundae for dessert. This is just real life.

"What really matters is what you do *most* of the time, not what you do occasionally. I call this the '80/20 approach': Do what you know you're supposed to 80% of the time; the other 20% of the time do whatever you want to! The idea is to take each of these areas seriously, but *not* to become a fanatic about any of them.

"I can give you an example in each of the three areas. Healthy self-empowerment starts with self-acceptance, which means that you have to start liking who you are. It *doesn't* mean you can't want to change some aspects of yourself, like your body weight. But if you can start by accepting who you are, your chances of reaching a reasonable goal are much greater.

"Likewise, we all know that exercise is important. Our bodies are designed to need activity. But, as you know from your experience, you can certainly overdo it. That's no better than not doing enough.

"And eating a sensible diet is essential for maintaining good health, not just a healthy body weight. But as Lucretius said thousands of years ago, 'One man's food is another man's poison.' There's no one, single dietary plan that's going to work for everybody. We all have different tastes. And as you also know from experience, it's important to have variety, good taste and an occasional splurge as part of your nutritional lifestyle."

That's just real life.

The Real-Life Difference

Are *you* beginning to see how real-life weight management differs from "old school" dieting? Before we start looking at each of the three areas in depth, let's take a look at how the three-part model redirects us from three obsolete dieting myths:

- The thinner you are, the better.
- Losing weight is mostly about food.
- Watch what you eat—*everything* you eat.

MYTH NO. 1: The Thinner You Are, the Better!

Because so much attention has been given to a "the thinner, the better" attitude, most programs have ultimately encouraged self-dissatisfaction and lowered self-esteem, exactly the opposite of what's needed. With what we now know about genetics and individual differences, there's no way that most people can become ultra-thin in a real-life, day-to-day situation.

This immense pressure to be thin has fostered a host of problems: poor body image, low self-esteem, eating disorders, fat prejudice. Unfortunately, even health professionals often contribute to the pressure by creating unrealistic expectations. How many people have been shamed by doctors or other health professionals for not falling neatly into a height-weight chart? How many people avoid doctors simply to avoid the embarrassment of the doctor's scales or scoldings?

The truth is that an individual's healthy weight is hard to define precisely. Like most things it depends on a number of factors, including genetics and perhaps even the individual's history of weight management attempts.

A reasonable goal is to get as healthy as you can, with body weight part of the mix, but you must enjoy your life in the process. If you don't, you certainly won't stay with whatever program you choose for long. You know full well that being at a healthy weight is an important part of overall health. But if you combine the pressure to lose weight with unrealistic goals, the outcome will likely be lower self-esteem and perhaps even disordered eating behaviors.

Real-life weight management places strong emphasis on self-empowerment and self-acceptance, in order to give you a solid foundation for staying motivated and making the permanent changes necessary to successfully adopt new habits. This is clearly the greatest challenge—as we know from the many people who succeed in losing weight initially, but are unable to integrate new habits permanently.

MYTH NO. 2: Losing Weight Is Mostly About Food

We have already discussed that the process of learning to live a healthy lifestyle and maintain a healthy weight involves much more than just what you put into your mouth. One of the most important keys that has been commonly undervalued is, without a doubt, *activity*. (I use the words *activity* and *exercise* interchangeably.) Today, research is showing us just how wrong it is to overlook the importance of activity. In maintaining weight loss, virtually no success factor is identified as strongly as regular, reasonably vigorous activity.

In the vast majority of past approaches, the emphasis on the need for activity (exercise) was either absent, or looked at more as an aside than as a critically important component. In fact, since activity is the only way to increase calorie burning above the number of calories you burn at rest, any effective long-term weight management program *has* to include physical activity.

You can certainly lose weight just by restricting calories. Your body's tendency to store or burn fat is basically determined by the balance between the number of calories you eat and the number of calories you burn. If you take in more calories than you burn, you'll gain weight. If you burn more than you take in, you'll lose weight.

"So," you might ask, "why don't I just quit eating? That's

a lot easier than having to get into an exercise program. Anyway, I don't like to exercise."

The problem is that when you lose weight just by dieting, some of the weight you lose comes from muscle. If you don't eat enough to fuel all of the processes your body has to perform every day just staying alive, the body converts some of the proteins in muscle to sugar (a type of carbohydrate) so it can make energy. Even though your body may have more than enough fat, it can't use just fat to make energy.

Exercise scientists have a saying, "Fat burns in the flame of sugar." This simply means that in order to use fat, in muscles for instance, the muscles must have an adequate supply of sugar. Since our body doesn't store very much carbohydrate, we have to replace it pretty much on a daily basis.

You generally don't want to lose muscle when you lose weight. In fact I often encourage clients to try to make *more* muscle. The key is activity.

You've probably heard and read lots of information about fat-burning and how such-and-such a product or program is a great fat-burner. But what's most important is that you burn enough calories on a regular basis to balance what you eat. You've just got to eat enough of the right kinds of foods (we'll get to this later!) to be able to lose weight as fat, not as fat and muscle.

Not surprisingly, some people have taken the calorie balance issue to extremes. (You will remember that's what Maggie did when she was in college.) The solution, as with most things, is moderation. Moderate activity is one of the three *main* components of real-life weight management—at least equal in importance to eating habits.

MYTH NO. 3: Watch What You Eat—Everything You Eat!

In addition to an almost exclusive emphasis on the dietary component of most typical weight management programs, in many cases the dietary suggestions are not only ineffective—they are unhealthy. Severe calorie restriction, meal replacements, fads, diet pills, magic formulations and high cost prepackaged meals are not eating styles most of us can adopt for very long.

I used to give clients scales and charts and meal records. We'd work out a detailed weekly meal plan. They'd record everything they ate, weigh and measure every portion.

Know what? Most of them would do it for a week or two, then it would become so tedious that the scales and charts went into the cupboard for good!

And in all honesty, I'd be the same way. Who has time to be that overwhelmed with the process of preparing and eating meals? Saving time is probably why prepackaged meals are so attractive to many people. The problem is that sooner or later—usually sooner—even the prepackaged meals become boring.

It's essential that you happily anticipate, for the most part, what you are going to eat. But like exercise and brushing your teeth, eating also doesn't *always* have to be fun; you do some things just because it's important to do them.

The bottom line is that you learn to plan and prepare meals that you look forward to eating. Reading labels and using the Food Guide Pyramid are crucial. We'll get to all that. But the most important point is that you don't get caught in an all-or-nothing approach to this area. If you say to yourself, "I'm never going to eat another candy bar as long as I live," you'll probably obsess on candy bars until you eat three at one time. Then you'll feel like you've blown your diet. Not necessary!

One additional piece of advice: Try not to think of your dietary habits in terms of "good" foods and "bad" foods. You'll only add fuel to the fire of that vicious lose-gain, success-failure spiral. Healthy eating is really more a matter of making sure that you give yourself enough of the right kind of foods on pretty much a regular basis. Think of your new dietary habits as something you can live with for the rest of your life. Some of it—the 80%—is eating what you know you need to. The other 20% is the stuff you eat without guilt, because it's fun and part of real-life eating.

"*So,*" you're probably wondering, "*are you telling me it's okay to eat an ice cream cone when I go to the mall?*"

Yeah, that's exactly what I'm saying. Just don't do it all the time. And be sure to eat some fruits and vegetables at some other time during the day!

Let's Get Started

That's the overview; now let's get started. For the rest of the book, we're going to take a look at each of the three components of real-life weight management one at a time, following how Maggie integrates them into her life and making plans for how you can implement them into your own life.

Jot down your answers to these self-assessment questions in each of the three areas. You may want to start a separate journal if you need more room. We will address your answers to these questions as we look at each area individually.

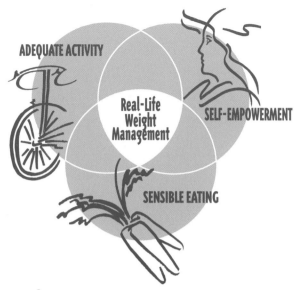

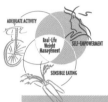

Self-Empowerment:

1. What are three things I like the most about myself?

_____

_____

_____

_____

2. Why do I feel I am ready to begin a new healthy lifestyle?

_____

_____

_____

_____

3. What qualities do I have that will help me succeed in achieving permanent change (i.e., patience, persistence, courage, etc.)? Do I have past experiences of successful change that can serve as a reminder of my capabilities?

_____

_____

_____

_____

_____

_____

Adequate Activity:

1. What are three things I can do to be more active on a daily basis (i.e., walking, stair climbing, yard work, etc.)?

_____

_____

_____

_____

2. What are the main roadblocks for me developing a regular exercise program?

_____

_____

_____

_____

3. What are three activities and/or types of exercise I enjoy enough to do on a regular basis?

_____

_____

_____

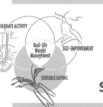

Sensible Eating:

1. What are my five favorite foods?

_____

_____

_____

_____

2. What are the three most difficult aspects I face with regard to eating an essentially healthy diet?

_____

_____

Section II. Real-Life Self-Empowerment
(Or, Dorothy, You've Had the Answer All Along)

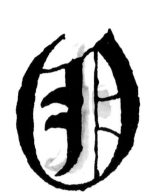nce upon a time, a young girl in Kansas named Dorothy (who looked remarkably like Judy Garland, a young girl in Hollywood who was already discovering the land of diet pills) found herself, through a circumstance of bad weather, in the wonderful land of Oz.

Once she got to Oz, all Dorothy really wanted to do was to get back home to Kansas. The Oz-ites told her there was one man in the land who had all the answers, and he called himself the Wizard. He lived in a giant green palace with a beauty salon and lots of cheap special effects.

On her way to Emerald City, where the Wizard lived, Dorothy picked up a scarecrow looking for a brain, a tin man looking for a heart, and a lion looking for courage—because they all believed the Wizard would have the magic answers to their problems, too.

When they found the wizard, he turned out to be a disappointing little blustery man behind a big curtain who had no magic after all. But he did have an important piece of information for Dorothy's virtue-seeking friends: he told them that they already had what they'd been looking for—they just didn't realize it.

A good witch who blew in on a bubble delivered pretty much the same message to Dorothy: Like the others, Dorothy didn't need a Wizard. She had the answer for how to get what she wanted all along.

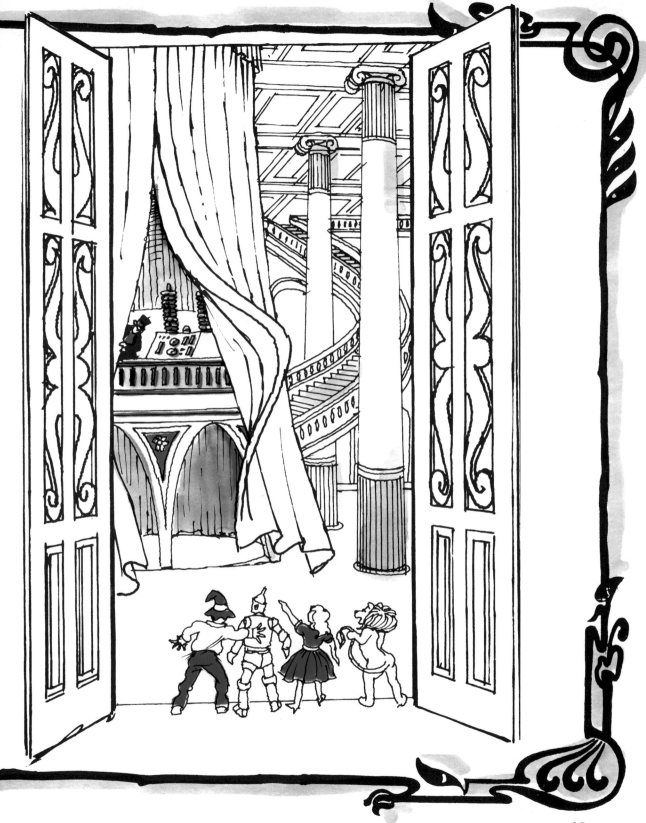

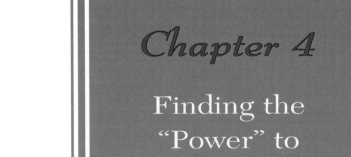

Chapter 4

Finding the "Power" to Stay Healthy

Real-life weight management isn't about just looking good. It's about getting healthy—getting healthy in our outlook as well as in our physical self. There is one important reason why you can't afford to undertake a weight management program without also taking a good look at your attitude about yourself, and at why you want to lose weight in the first place. That reason is simple: Weight management programs generally don't fail because people don't know *how to lose weight* in the first place—they fail because people don't know *how to stay motivated* to maintain their healthy living habits.

Since practicing healthy habits is essentially about taking care of ourselves, we need to start with our attitude about ourselves.

I use the term "self-empowerment" in a broad sense—to cover all those qualities that will give you the strength, commitment and power to create a healthy lifestyle and stick with it. No one can give you this power (not even the diet gurus), but you can develop it on your own—just as Dorothy found that she had the power to get back to Kansas on her own, and her friends found that they already had the heart, the intelligence and the courage they needed.

In fact, you will probably find that on the yellow brick road to a healthy weight and a healthy lifestyle, you will need to rely on your own heart, intelligence and courage even more than on food and exercise plans. Self-empowerment is about finding these qualities in ourselves and using them to reach our goals.

In the next four chapters we're going to look at some issues which are often related to self-empowerment in the weight management process: self-acceptance, body image, healthy weight, and managing the stresses of everyday living. These will give you a place to start in your own self-acceptance journey. But it is just a start—don't stop here.

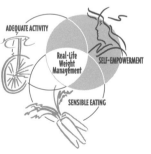

There's no way one book can cover all of the issues in detail, unless it's an encyclopedia! There are many valuable resources available—more than ever before—that can help you find and develop ways to like who you are. You might want to try counseling and support group approaches, or books, tapes and videos. (See the Resources list at the end of this book.)

Empowering Yourself With Self-Acceptance

"Accept yourself for who you are." How many times have you heard that? Probably too many! But knowing that's what you *should* do, and actually *doing* it are two different things. In fact, accepting yourself can be a very difficult task—especially if you have been getting other messages for years.

Weight management often has been pitched as learning to change the things you dislike about yourself. Unfortunately, this prevailing attitude is like any self-fulfilling prophecy— it's created a lot of people who are focused on disliking themselves (Maggie, for example).

This linking of health and appearance, and the resulting self-discontent, has not resulted in a positive change in weight management. As I've mentioned, during the last 10 years the average weight among men and women has increased by about 10 pounds.

Could it be that it just isn't in human nature to sustain efforts based on self-dislike? Efforts founded in a negative state of mind often seem to bring negative results. Researchers, and common sense, tell us that one of the most important ingredients for bringing about true behavior change is feeling good about who we are to begin with.

"But," I can hear Maggie saying, *"if I liked who I was at this weight, I wouldn't need a weight management program!"*

You might be thinking the same thing, since you've been taught to analyze and criticize your body as if you were doing a Siskel & Ebert movie review. But now is a great time to start shifting into a new pattern of thinking—self-acceptance, and ultimately, self-empowerment. This is the first and perhaps most important part of the real-life triad, at least in the long run.

Sure, activity and sensible eating habits are extremely important. But either or both probably won't work unless you accept the idea that weight management is just the natural extension of your wanting to be as nice to yourself as possible because you care about yourself and want to take responsibility for your health.

That's right—the whole thing is about you liking you, just the way you are.

"So you mean I have to stop criticizing my body like a bad movie and start enjoying it, exactly the way it is right now?" asks Maggie.

From the look on her face, I can tell she thinks I'm a little crazy! But the answer is, Yes. A lot of people seem to prefer the "If…, then…" approach to self-acceptance. "If I lose 30 pounds, then I'll treat myself to…" or "If I fit into those jeans from three years ago, then I'll go out and dance the way I used to…."

The problem with "If…, then…" is that you're stuck in a holding pattern, not feeling good about yourself and waiting for magic to strike. But change rarely happens while we're stuck in a rut!

Pleasure Not Punishment

For many of us, the idea of giving ourselves healthy food and enjoyable activity sounds more like work (or punishment!) than kindness or pleasure. That's often because we don't have much practice at self-care. For those of us who aren't ready to change our food preparation, shopping, eating or activity habits, the best place to start is by practicing small acts of self-care. We'll talk more specifically about these shortly.

Of course, self-acceptance alone won't get you optimum health or a healthy body weight. But it clearly sets the stage. It provides the strong foundation to gradually make the changes you want. Just look at the popular examples of celebrities like Oprah Winfrey and Susan Powter, who have both emphasized the essential link between self-acceptance and successful weight management in their own lives.

Popular author Deepak Chopra, MD, expresses it this way in the very first lines of his book, *Perfect Weight*, "Instead of beginning with the assumption that there's something wrong with you that needs to be corrected, our starting point here is the idea that there's nothing essentially wrong with you at all…. If you've been trying hard to live up to an artificial, media-generated notion of what the human body should look like, it's easy to forget that powerful forces of nature worked for millions of years to create you exactly as you are. Your body is a miracle of biological engineering."

This "miracle of engineering" needs to be taken care of just like any good machine—better, in fact, because we are so much more complex than mere machines. We all take better care of the things we like and appreciate than we do of the things we don't like, at least most of the time. Self-acceptance is just a part of taking care of yourself, from the inside out.

Question Check-Back

In Chapter 3, you wrote down the three things you like the most about yourself. Do any of them have to do with your physical appearance? Or do they have more to do with what you value?

Practicing Self-Acceptance

We will be doing a number of written exercises in this chapter. Let's begin with this simple one.

Exercise No.1

Write down the three things you value the most in your life.

_____

_____

_____

Your Values and Your Health

The practice of self-acceptance really involves identifying fundamental values for the process of managing your health, including your body weight. After you've identified your values, the next step is to find ways to connect your healthy living efforts to what is most important to you.

For example, let's say one of your values is your family. How will a healthier lifestyle impact your family? Will you have more energy to enjoy your family life? Will you be a better role model for your children? Will feeling good about your body weight make you a more pleasant person to be around?

Let's take another example. Imagine that one of your values is a spiritual one. How will healthy living impact your spiritual life? Does taking good care of yourself, body and mind, align with your beliefs about your spiritual responsibility? Will you be better able to carry out a higher purpose in life if you are as healthy as possible?

An example of something on my value list is "self-worth." I can connect my lifestyle habits to this value with the statement: "I place a high value on taking good care of my health because I am a worthwhile person who deserves to be cared for in the best possible way."

Question Check-Back

Look back at your answer to question 6 in Chapter 2. You may find that until now your weight management efforts have been based on values you don't really, deep down, believe in. (No wonder so many of us have had a hard time sticking with the effort!)

Now contrast that statement with this one: "I place a high value on weight control because I don't think my looks are acceptable as they are."

Which statement has more *lasting* value?

Your values are really the foundation of your weight management efforts.

You may realize that you have been trying to lose weight based on the belief that thin people are more attractive. But do you really believe that the attractiveness of people is based on body weight? Do you believe that attractiveness is an exterior or an interior quality? What makes another person attractive to you?

In *Fat Is a Feminist Issue*, author Susan Orbach discusses in length another common example of a belief behind many attempts to lose weight—the belief that "women need to be thin to appeal to men." Most advertising certainly paints that picture. But this expectation may conflict with your own belief that women should not have to conform to impossible ideals (or body sizes!) to please anyone.

Here are some questions for you to answer. You may discover that the beliefs at the heart of your weight control efforts are in serious conflict with your true value system. Your weight management efforts will have a much better chance of succeeding if they are based on what you truly believe is important in life.

Exercise No. 2

1. What is more important, good looks or good relationships?

_____

_____

_____

2. Do the people I really care about love me because of the way I look, or because of the way I am?

_____

_____

_____

3. Who are the people I most admire? Is it because of the way they look or something else?

_____

_____

_____

4. It has taken me a long time to get my body to where it is right now. Can I accept that changing its appearance is a slow process?

_____

_____

_____

Tell It to My Thighs!

"Yeah, right, tell all this value stuff to my thighs," chimes Maggie. "I still want to look good when I go to my reunion. It *is* important to me. I'll feel better about myself if I do. Isn't that okay?"

For the short term, that may be okay. But in the long run, Maggie may be sabotaging her success. If looking good was such a great incentive for her, why hasn't it worked so far? Maggie probably needs to try some new ways of thinking if she's going to be able to get and keep new habits, and the new body to go with it. She will have a much better chance of losing the weight she needs to if she begins the process by feeling good about herself *right now*.

That way she won't be constantly looking into the future for the time when it'll be okay to feel good about herself. (Because real trouble sets in when the weight comes off and we find we *still* don't feel good about ourselves! And the "trouble" can show up in regained weight.)

You're not alone in your quest to discover your values. We're seeing an increasing emphasis on a return to values, demonstrated in the popularity of books such as Steven Covey's *The Seven Principles of Highly Effective People* and William Bennett's *Book of Virtues*.

Twelve-step programs, like the original one developed for Alcoholics Anonymous, can be found for almost any desired behavior change, from Overeaters Anonymous to Gamblers Anonymous to Shoppers Anonymous. They all, like the original, encourage and reinforce the development of spiritual principles to be practiced in all of our affairs. That's just another way of saying that your lifestyle—including how you take care of your health—should be based on your values, not the external pressures of the media or the mirror.

The next three exercises will help you get started on creating the healthy self-acceptance that leads to self-empowerment.

Answer the following questions, using your own values as a foundation:

Exercise No. 3

1. Write three reasons why practicing a healthy lifestyle is important to you?

_____

_____

_____

_____

2. Write three reasons why getting and keeping a healthy body weight is important?

_____

_____

_____

_____

3. Based on what you've read so far, write a list of old ideas about weight loss that you no longer want to keep, and replace them with new ideas that you would like to live by. (Even if you're not sure about them yet, write them down.)

_____

_____

_____

_____

_____

Exercise No. 4

1. Write a list of things that give you pleasure. Include everything you can think of. Be imaginative; think back to enjoyments you may have forgotten. (The longer the list, the better.)

_____

_____

_____

_____

_____

Exercise No. 4 – continued

2. Start planning ways to include more of these "pleasure-givers" in your life. Schedule them on your daily planner. Put them on your refrigerator. Maybe it's "Go to a movie at least once week," or "Take a camping trip in the spring," or "Take a nap on Sundays," or "Call Jane in Pittsburgh." They can be simple (bubble baths) or complex (learn a new language). If the pleasure-giver is a certain kind of food, don't worry—we'll plan it into your eating habits. But you will find that your list of pleasures probably goes far beyond food!

3. Remember that you are doing these things for yourself because *it is healthy* to feel pleasure! (Read *Healthy Pleasures* by David Sobel and Robert Ornstein, if you need to be convinced!) You are also learning the art of being good to yourself. If you start to feel guilty or selfish, call someone support-ive who will set you straight!

One good way to boost your self-esteem is to take the time to do good deeds. (Just be careful that you don't do so many good deeds for others that you forget it is also your responsibility to do good deeds for yourself whenever possible.)

Exercise No. 5

1. For one week, every morning write down three nice things that you have done for other people the day before. (These can be anything from smiling at a stranger on the street to babysitting for a friend for a weekend.)

_____

_____

_____

_____

_____

_____

_____

_____

2. For the next week, plan three nice things you are going to do each day.

_____

_____

_____

_____

_____

_____

_____

_____

_____

3. Write a list of nice things you would like to do regularly. (These can include being more supportive of your spouse, being less cranky at work, complimenting your children more, etc.)

_____

_____

_____

_____

_____

Not an Overnight Sensation

Self-acceptance is a tall order. Behavior change is one of the most difficult challenges there is. That's why health practices (not just weight management) that are so important are so difficult for many of us to stick to. After a lifetime of peering in the mirror for flaws, one thing is for sure: You're probably not going to wake up tomorrow morning feeling overjoyed at the prospect of living in your perfect body for another 24 hours!

Self-acceptance is a *lifelong* process. Some days you will undoubtedly feel better about yourself than others. That's okay. The process takes commitment and courage (more values), because even when so many things around you are hinting that you should be dissatisfied with who you are, you need the strength to believe in your own conviction that you're really okay. Practice, as with everything else, makes all the difference.

You've already written down three of your most important values. You can undoubtedly identify many more. Once you've identified your self-acceptance beliefs, it's just a matter of practicing them over and over again. Just as your muscles get stronger when you stay with a regular activity routine, your self-acceptance muscles will get stronger when you take up liking yourself on a regular basis!

Remember that trying to take care of yourself out of...

> **Hatred**—"I hate fat!"
> **Judgment**—"I look so awful. No one would go out with someone who looks like me."
> **Fear**—"No one will like me if I don't lose weight."

or

Control—"I will never allow myself to look like that."

…is a long, difficult, and seldom successful road.

The more you like yourself, the easier it will be to stay motivated to practice the healthy living habits which reflect your value system. Because you'll be doing it out of love. And everyone knows that love is the strongest motivator there is!

I suggest you avoid any weight management program or counselor that makes you feel guilty or ashamed of your behaviors or your appearance. What you should get is support for your unique and valuable self—no matter what your size, no matter how "bad" you think your behaviors are.

Real-life weight management isn't a program. It's a lifelong process. And self-acceptance is an integral part.

Self-Acceptance: Ten Tips for Your Journey

Here are some other thoughts to guide you in the self-acceptance process:

1. **Self-acceptance does not mean denial.** It doesn't mean pretending that you're not at health risk if you are, pretending that walking to your car to go to work is adequate activity for your health, pretending that your food choices are healthy if they are not. Self-acceptance is facing these facts (not moral weaknesses) and still liking yourself, flaws and all. And when you face these facts, you can appreciate that you're doing the best that you can at the moment. It's much easier to pay closer attention to your behaviors and motivations—and to decide on effective ways to help you make changes—when you start with compassion for yourself rather than condemnation. It certainly works better when dealing with others.

2. **Self-acceptance is not a "cure-all" for eating problems.** While self-acceptance is an integral part of the process of recovering from eating disorders, most experts agree that enhanced self-esteem alone will not make an eating disorder disappear. Accepting that you may have a problem, without self-blame, is often the first step in changing that behavior—but it's not the only step.

3. **Self-acceptance is not an excuse not to act.** It doesn't mean "anything goes!" Remember the 80/20 principle? Self-acceptance means doing what you know you need to 80% of the time. The Serenity Prayer says it very well: "Grant me the serenity to accept the things I cannot change, the courage to change the things I can, and the wisdom to know the difference." Self-acceptance is not a question of control. Rather, it's accepting that there are things you cannot control—like your genetics. But with courage you can change other things. Gaining "the wisdom to know the difference" is the real key. In your ongoing self-discovery process you will likely find some surprises—some things you thought you could change but can't, and vice versa.

4. **It's never too late to start.** In fact, the longer you've lived, the more experience you've probably had in learning to accept who you are!

5. **Self-acceptance comes differently for everybody.** River rafting may be just the ticket for helping your best friend learn to accept her tomboy side, while a monthly massage for relaxation and body awareness may be more what you need. Kelly Brownell, PhD, in *The LEARN Program for Weight Control* describes two different types of changers: "solo" and "social" changers. One of the first steps in your self-acceptance journey is to identify which type you are and accept it as okay. Solo changers are highly independent, and don't like to discuss much of their behavior change with others. Social changers like to talk about their process with others, and often choose to join groups of like-minded individuals. In either case, the support of others seems to be very helpful for almost everyone. Solo changers may do much better working with a personal trainer. Social changers would find group

activity sessions or support group meetings helpful. Solo changers may still enjoy group sessions—they'll just be quieter during the meetings!

6. **Patience is paramount in practicing self-acceptance.** There's no rush. Patience and persistence are just as important in developing self-acceptance as they are in weight management and health management. We're talking months, years and decades here—not days and weeks! As an infant you probably liked yourself just fine. The attention to, and effects of, the mirror's feedback didn't come until later. Regaining that perspective you had as an infant is going to take awhile. So settle in for the long haul.

7. **One useful technique for self-acceptance is acting "as if."** You may be waiting forever if you decide to wait for a mood of overwhelming self-love to envelope you. The patience/persistence part doesn't mean just waiting, it means planning and choosing attitudes and behaviors that demonstrate self-acceptance and self-care. Acting "as if" you are a person with a great capacity to nurture and care for yourself may well be the first step to becoming that person.

8. **Your self-acceptance journey is likely to have high points and low points, big jumps forward and surprise setbacks.** What works one month may not work the next. Don't belittle yourself for this reality. Allow yourself to travel the self-acceptance path at your own pace. Trust your instincts for what will work best. But don't let yourself think you've failed if you find yourself in some familiar self-critical mood. Just recognize it and try to get back on the path. A good periodic test is to ask yourself, "Am I taking this action out of appreciation and caring for myself—or for some other reason?" Or, "Would I recommend this behavior to someone I love (my child, for example)?"

9. **The rewards of self-acceptance are endless!** It's because you are improving the most important and lasting human relationship you'll ever have—the one with yourself! There seems to be fairly unanimous

agreement among experts that in most any situation you're able to give more to others when you first take care of yourself. And the first step in taking care of yourself is to accept yourself for who you are.

10. **You get a Free Gift!** The gift of self-acceptance is that you are going to find it easier to accept others. You will likely end up being an even nicer person than you are right now! You may find this as much or more rewarding than reaching your goal weight.

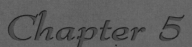

Chapter 5

Maggie's Image of Maggie

Maggie has spent most of her adult life trying to be size 8. That is her dream size. She remembers magic times when she actually could fit into a size 8; and she remembers the disappointment of having to give away her size 8 jeans when she just couldn't fit into them anymore (and boy how she tried!). She can't help but feel that if she were just a size 8 again, somehow she would feel so much better about herself….

And, of course, Maggie's husband, Jim, lays awake at night thinking about what it would be like if only Maggie could fit into a size 8.

When Maggie's children think about their mother, they think to themselves, "Mom's great, but we'd love her even more if she were a size 8."

Huh? Of course Maggie's husband and children do *not* stay awake nights or love her any less for not being a size 8—they love her for who she is. Her size is important only when they buy her something for her birthday or Christmas. (Unfortunately, in some cases this may not always be the case. Spouses, significant others and even children sometimes do contribute to the feelings of guilt and shame associated with unsuccessful weight loss attempts. Hopefully, this isn't true in your situation. If it is, it clearly becomes a reality you have to address on your journey to self-acceptance.)

In Maggie's case, it is more likely that her extreme devotion to being a size 8 is affecting her family in a more negative way than her actual size ever could. Jim gets frustrated that he must continually reassure Maggie that she looks fine to him. The kids find it hard to understand why Mom seems to sometimes be depressed without any apparent reason.

Maggie's dissatisfaction and unhappiness with herself, coupled with her fantasies about how life would be "If only..." frequently interfere with her and her family's ability to enjoy life and each other's company.

It's easy to lose our perspective on body image. Focusing on clothing sizes, numbers on the bathroom scale, the imagined shape of the body in general and specific body parts can lead us to believe that these things are all more important in the scheme of things than they really are.

Before I go any farther, let me reemphasize that developing a healthy body image does not mean ignoring the important health risks and consequences that can accompany being overweight. There is no question that obesity increases the risk of developing a number of diseases—diabetes, hypertension, certain cancers, heart disease, joint problems.

Having a healthy body image simply means that the best place to start any process of taking care of ourselves (including managing our weight) is to look at ourselves with honesty and compassion, rather than with distortion and blame.

A healthy body image encourages an honest recognition of the possible need to lose some weight. If you take a real-life, self-styled, one-small-change-at-a-time, long-term approach to improving how you feel about your body, you're not just going to help your weight management efforts—you're going to add a new dimension of greater enjoyment of your life.

And that couldn't hurt at any size, right?

Repeat After Me: There's No Such Thing!

Perhaps the biggest weight management "naked truth" of them all is related to body image: There is no such thing as a perfect body. Just ask any model, actress, fitness professional or exercise video star—or any photographer who touches up celebrity photos! Visit the set of an exercise video in production and you may be amazed to see that far more time can be spent making sure that make-up and wardrobe are near perfect than is spent in doing the exercise program.

We *all* see our own imperfections, and often imagine that everyone else sees them, too. Self-acceptance and a healthy body image are certainly very much interconnected. As much as we might want to believe in a model of perfection that we should strive for, in reality perfection is an illusion. It has little bearing on real-life weight management. The truth about our naked selves—including our bodies—is that we are all humanly imperfect. And that's okay.

Let's take a look at these factors which will help you determine how best to pursue the development of a healthy body image:

- Finding the approach that works for you
- Recognizing and resisting cultural messages
- Reflecting on your own body image history
- Replacing old thinking and habits with new thinking and habits

The Approach That Works For You

Let me mention at the outset that while all of us have varying degrees of satisfaction with our bodies, more serious body image issues can accompany eating disorders (anorexia, bulimia, binge eating) and/or a variety of other psychological issues. These require specialized help beyond the scope of this book. If this may be part of your situation, your first step is to seek a qualified counseling professional to help you determine your needs.

It's important that you see that your body image attitudes are personal and unique to you. The solutions that work best will be the ones that match your personal style and needs. There are books and tapes, support groups and professional counselors that all discuss the issue of body image. *There is no one best way to cultivate a healthy body image.* What works for you might not work for someone else, and vice versa. And what works for you today might not work tomorrow.

In the next few pages, we'll look at some approaches you might consider for enhancing your body image. If none of these feels right, seek out others. As with all aspects of real-life health and weight management, two factors are key to your success:

1. Self-knowledge—exploring your own feelings, beliefs and behaviors

2. Self-responsibility—recognizing that you have a choice

Fighting Cultural Messages

It's easy to see how our culture feeds unhealthy body image attitudes. Movies, television, magazines, billboards all reinforce the idea that what we look like is extremely important. And not just with regard to weight management issues. "Regain your youth, attractiveness and self-confidence," proclaim the multitude of hair replacement ads which populate the pages of most any daily newspaper.

Psychologists Foreyt and Goodrick report that in 1992 there were 620,000 cosmetic surgeries that were performed in the United States for purely appearance reasons. A 1987 Harris poll reported that 96% of Americans wanted to change something about their bodies. Talk about an obsession with appearance!

But there is one answer to all the hype that is seldom discussed, and it's this: Question what you see and hear! Ask yourself, "Do I really believe this is true? Do I really believe this is necessary?"

It's amazing how easy it is to forget that we do have a choice.

Sure, it would be great if the predominant media messages started changing right now, telling us that being healthy is what really matters, not how we look; that everyone has his or her own unique inner beauty; that there is no one way everyone should look. But you and I both know that there's too much invested for that change to happen quickly. It's starting to happen, but it's going to take some time to turn the tide on the media's portrayal of body image.

The good news is you don't have to wait! If you want to, you can start accepting yourself and how your body looks today. Then, if you want or need to change some aspect—like body weight—you can do it based on an honest recognition that you value your health, that you're making a change because you care about yourself, believe in yourself, and respect yourself (not because the media is telling you to!).

Looking Back: Your Body Image History

Media images are just one of the ways you might have picked up unrealistic, distorted ideas about body image. Family, friends, coworkers and other people in your life might have influenced how you feel about the way you look. Maggie was teased by her classmates in school. Perhaps your mother was always concerned about her weight, or your father pressured you with his beliefs about the ideal size for you to be.

One technique that can help you understand your own ideas about body image is to find a quiet place and write a brief history of how you have felt about your body throughout your life—during childhood, the teenage years, young adulthood, middle age, etc. Take note of what was happening at various times in your life when you felt especially positive or negative about your body. You can use photographs to help jog your memory.

The goal here is not to blame anyone for anything—most especially not to blame yourself in any way ("Grant me the serenity to accept the things I cannot change..."). The idea is to build your self-knowledge, so that you have the tools to change your body image beliefs if such a change can make you more healthy.

Writing this history takes a commitment of time on your part, and it may bring back some not-so-pleasant memories. But you will gain valuable information about the role body image has played in your life. You might discover where some of your old beliefs were formed and the effects they have had. Try to pay special attention to the connection between how you felt about your body and how you felt about yourself in general.

Depending on your unique history, you might discover that your beliefs about body image are connected to other beliefs about family and relationships, men and women in general, power and control, physical safety, sexuality, separation or grief, success and failure, and more. It's amazing how much power we can give to the idea of body size and shape!

Replacing the Old With the New

I asked Maggie to do a brief exercise (originating from eating disorders educator and author Becky Jackson) to help create new awareness about her body image ideas. "Maggie, you once asked me how you can figure out what your beliefs are today about body image," I suggested. "Here's an exercise that will help."

"Write the words *fat*, *thin*, *big*, and *small* on a sheet of paper, leaving space between the words. Then, one at a time, consider each word and write down other words or phrases that automatically come into your head when you think of that particular word. Do it quickly, and don't censor yourself—just write what pops up into your mind."

Fat _____

_____

_____

Thin _____

_____

_____

Big _____

_____

_____

Small _____

_____

"How will doing this help me to understand my feelings about how I look?" asked Maggie.

"It's just part of the process of increasing your self-knowledge," I told her. "This exercise will give you a personal look at some of the associations you have with body size. It's important information about yourself."

"Okay," Maggie thinks to herself, and writes...

> **Fat**—weak, ugly, failure...
> **Thin**—success, pretty, clothes...
> **Big**—me, hopeless, forever...
> **Small**—I wish, happy, proud...

Maggie apparently doesn't think big and fat are so hot—small and thin are her dreams.

What words come to your mind when you do this exercise? They will give you an idea about your beliefs. Once you've identified these beliefs, you can start to change them with two steps:

1. being aware of the "old ideas" when they show up in your head

2. replacing them with your "new ideas" for body image

Now, how do your find your new ideas? That's easy—you choose them! Remember, I told you that you have a choice about what you want to believe. Also remember that these beliefs are uniquely yours.

Here are some examples of old ideas and new ideas. You can write your own comparisons on the next page based on the words you wrote for *fat*, *thin*, *big* and *small*.

My Old Beliefs	My New Beliefs
Being fat is a sign of weakness (or stupidity, laziness, etc.).	Being fat is a physical condition, and does not signify strength or weakness.
Thinness represents success (or willpower, beauty, etc).	I do not judge people's personal qualities based on size.

Be careful here! You may find that you have some old beliefs that surprise you. For example:

Fat people are happy and fun to be with.	My enjoyment of people does not depend on how they look.
Thin people are weak and sickly.	Health and vigor are not determined by body size.

My Old Beliefs	My New Beliefs

Here's another one from Becky Jackson's workshops that you may want to consider: Write down the word *average* and see what other words pop into your head.

Average _____

You may find that you have spent so much time trying to place yourself at the extremes of fat or thin, big or small, that you never really thought about what it might mean to be somewhere in the middle, or average!

Our culture seldom teaches that it's okay to be average, even though the truth is that in one way or another that's exactly what we all are. We have our strengths and weaknesses, our positive and negative qualities, our successes and failures, our ups and downs—and so do our bodies. Most of it adds up to each of us being unique, individual, special selves— above average in some ways and below average in others (for me that's being able to draw a picture better than my 5-year-old!).

Ultimately we're all wonderfully one-of-a-kind, imperfect humans. Expecting our bodies to live up to unrealistic stan- dards is often a sad result of not being able to accept the truth about our very special, very unique, but imperfect humanness.

You may want to create old and new beliefs about the concept of average, too. Here's an example:

Old	New
Being average is boring.	It's okay for me to be average.

The important thing in this exercise is that you take the time to create your own list of old and new beliefs about body size. And it probably won't match anyone else's list—it doesn't have to.

Those New Beliefs

When you're working on your list of new beliefs about body image and body size, be sure to write some that specifically have to do with *your* body. For instance:

Old	New
I will be able to love my body when I'm size _____.	I accept and love my body at the size it is today.
My body is not as beautiful as many other people's bodies.	My body is beautiful exactly as it is because it's uniquely mine.
Other people probably don't find my body pleasing.	People love me for who I am as a whole person, NOT for my body size.

Perhaps most important in creating your new list of body image values is this key point: You are not *just* your body. You are a complex emotional, mental, spiritual and physical being, of which your body size and shape is only *one part*.

You may very well discover in creating new ideas to replace old beliefs that you have had a tendency to place much more importance on body size and shape than is realistic. Most of us have—it's certainly the message we are constantly bombarded with. If so, you've now discovered more very important information about yourself, and you need to ask yourself one more important question:

"If I were not unhappy and dissatisfied with my body, is there something else I would be unhappy and dissatisfied with?"

Preoccupation with how you look, with your body weight and shape, clothing size, etc., may be a comfortable habit you've developed to avoid looking at more significant areas of your life that may need attention, such as your self-esteem, or how satisfied you are with your relationships or your work.

You may discover that you have spent too much time focused on how you look and too little time focusing on who you really are and what you really need to be happy and fulfilled in your life.

In real-life weight management, numbers on the scale, clothing sizes and prejudices that are associated with various body types are of little importance. But finding out and accepting who you really are (including your body) is *very important*. Why? Because you will never be able to take care of yourself in a healthy way if you don't like yourself *right now*, or if you don't know yourself very well. It just won't happen.

"But I still want to lose some weight!" exclaims Maggie. "I think I'm beginning to understand what you're talking about. I can look in the mirror and appreciate my body. But I still want to change it. Isn't that okay?"

"Of course it is, Maggie. Developing a healthy body image is simply opening a door. It frees you from the traps and pressures of constantly comparing yourself with some mythical image of what you think you're supposed to look like. Once you can accept what you look like right now, you'll be much more likely to adapt your lifestyle to include adequate activity and sensible eating habits. And since you accept yourself for who you are and what you look like one day at time, you'll also feel good about whatever happens to your body size and weight down the road, no matter what the results. That's how self-acceptance, activity and sensible eating all work together."

What Does Good Body Image Look Like?

What would it feel like to be someone with a "good" body image? Here are some possibilities. Remember, these are totally individual. Write down your own list (these are just my ideas) of what it would feel and look like to have a healthy body image—and then begin acting as though you already do!

- I accept my body size (no matter what it is) as uniquely beautiful because it is a part of me.

- I do my best to be caring and nurturing of my body, as I would for anything I love.

- I know that other people are much more than their bodies, and I don't make judgments about them based on body size or shape.

- I don't expect my body to be perfect. I allow myself and others to be comfortably average rather than rating on a scale of fat/thin, big/small, good/bad extremes.

- When I see and hear media and social messages that imply that there is something wrong with my body because of the way it looks, I am able to separate the outside, superficial values from my own deeper, personal values.

• I am able to view my body objectively and accurately, without judging or attaching a moral value.

• I enjoy a respectful, loving partnership with my body, rather than feeling a need to fight, control or force my body in any way.

• I know that my body is much more than an object to be viewed, and I deeply appreciate the many capabilities and talents of my body that have nothing to do with how I appear to others.

• I recognize the health issues associated with my body, and I pursue solutions if there are concerns—because I am taking care of myself.

• When I find myself feeling negative about my body, I explore my feelings about what is going on in my life to discover if there are other areas that are bothering me.

• When I find myself feeling negative about my body, I identify the old beliefs that are surfacing and replace them with new beliefs. (It gets easier the more I practice!)

• I am able to forgive myself for the times when I have not chosen the healthiest behaviors for myself.

• I am able to celebrate positive things I do for my body, even small things.

• I recognize that my body is a dramatic and responsive machine, and I am optimistic that my relationship with my body will only get better over time.

More Ideas for Healthy Body Image

Here are some other ideas to think about as you work through the process of developing a healthy body image:

- Try to view yourself in a mirror as a whole person, rather than as a collection of parts.

- Explore touch for connection, healing or pleasure, with methods such as massage or other forms of bodywork.

- Experiment with relaxation methods, such as breathing techniques and meditation.

- Develop an appreciation of your senses through greater awareness of music, art and nature.

- Get in touch with your body sensations during physical activities you enjoy (gardening, walking, dancing, cycling, whatever).

- Take good care of all aspects of your body—teeth, hair, eyes, skin….

- Seek out people who are positive and nonjudgmental about their own appearance and the appearance of others.

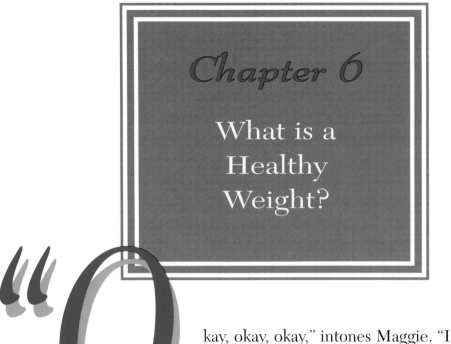

Chapter 6

What is a Healthy Weight?

"Okay, okay, okay," intones Maggie. "I think I really am beginning to understand that wearing a size 8 is a bit unrealistic. And I know that what I look like in the mirror shouldn't be my only motivation to lose weight. I recognize that it's a health issue. And I want to get more healthy.

"But I've also been told time and again that it's important to have some goal weight in mind, or else I won't have anything to shoot for. Almost every program I've ever tried has weighed me every time I went to a session. Or I've been pinched and measured to be able to get some prediction for how much I should weigh. So, what's the deal? Can you tell me how much I should weigh?"

"I can only give you an estimate," I tell her. "As with most things, there are many of factors, like your genetics and your history, which have a lot of influence on a reasonable goal. But I also know that in real life people do want to have some kind of an idea of what a reasonable goal is for them. The truth is, with the hugely important first step of self-acceptance becoming a part of your everyday life, your attention to adequate activity and sensible eating will ultimately determine what you will weigh.

"To me, the most important goal of a weight management lifestyle is to reduce your risk of health problems. As you just said, that's the key to understanding the seeming paradox between accepting yourself (and your body) for who you are right now and still wanting to make some physical changes to become healthier. They aren't contradictory feelings. They're integrally related.

"The good news is that researchers are discovering that even a modest reduction in weight can have tremendous health benefits, especially for those with weight-related health problems, such as high blood pressure, diabetes, or osteoarthritis, which may be caused or aggravated by their weight. Regardless of the starting weight, losing just 10-15% of it will improve health; it doesn't matter where the starting weight is. And that's the key."

Number Magic

Maggie's interest in a number for how much she should weigh is certainly not unique. I'd like to have a nickel for each time someone in the United States steps on a scale! And I've definitely done my share of measuring people with skinfold calipers, tape measures and underwater weighing tanks to estimate a healthy weight. But I've learned some really interesting things over the years:

- Your healthy weight might be what you are right now!

- Suggesting a **healthy weight range** is preferable to giving a suggested ideal body weight. There are so many individual factors involved that it is usually better to suggest a range of weight as a goal, rather than one specific number. We don't live in an ideal world! Why create unrealistic goals?

- The issue in real-life weight management is empowering you to take care of yourself, not strengthening the shackles of control often associated with focusing on some future scale number.

From Simple to Complex

With these ideas in mind, let's look at a few of the most common ways to establish a body weight goal. I'll certainly point out the ones I prefer in different situations!

There are many different techniques for estimating a given individual's healthy weight range. Some require expertise and training in doing the estimation; others are pretty straightforward. Let me start with the easiest techniques. Then I'll address some of the more technical methods, for those of you who might be interested.

The "Weight for a Year" Method

One straightforward method recommended by K. D. Brownell and T. A. Wadden in a 1991 scientific report is to shoot for the lowest weight that you've been able to maintain for at least one straight year since age 21. The assumption is that if you've been able to maintain this weight for at least a year, it probably wasn't the result of a crash diet or an unmanageable exercise program.

Maggie, for example, was able to maintain a weight of about 140 pounds for a little longer than a year. So, that's one reasonable goal weight for her. We can create a healthy range simply by saying that between about 138 and 142 pounds is reasonable.

What's the lowest weight you've been able to comfortably maintain for at least one straight year since you were 21?

The Lose 10–15% of Current Weight Method

Without doing any measurements, simply subtract 10% and 15% of your current weight as a healthy range for weight loss. Former Surgeon General C. Everett Koop, who launched the "Shape Up America" program in the fall of 1994, emphasized that the gradual loss of even a relatively small amount of weight can have immediate health benefits.

While this method is probably most appropriate for those who have weight-related health problems such as high blood pressure, diabetes, osteoarthritis, etc., it can be used by anyone. From a medical perspective, a clinical diagnosis of obesity, which often leads to these and other health problems, is usually described as being more than 20% above your healthy weight.

But, as we all need to remember, healthy weight is a totally individual proposition! This method simply suggests that if you have weight-related health concerns, you don't have to lose 20% of your weight to improve your health. Just a modest weight reduction can have huge benefits.

Since Maggie's weight is about 20% higher than her healthy weight, let's use her as an example. Maggie weighs 160 pounds, so this method estimates that a range for her would be to lose between 16 (10%) and 24 (15%) pounds. Subtracting these values from her current weight, we'd estimate a healthier weight range of between 136 and 144 pounds.

In Maggie's case this method estimated a range pretty darn close to the one based on her one-year maintenance weight. This won't always be true.

You can fill in the following blanks to determine your weight range based on losing 10-15% of your current weight:

Current weight = _____pounds

Current weight x .10 = _____ pounds (10% loss)

Current weight x .15 = _____pounds (15% loss)

(Current weight) - (10% loss) = _____pounds

(Current weight) - (15% loss) = _____pounds

The healthy weight range you just figured out might be higher than you had in mind! Remember that it's just an estimation. And don't become so focused on this range that you let those old control thoughts creep back in! If you have weight-related health problems, reaching this range means you've dramatically improved your health.

Using a Formula

For those women (sorry guys!) who are interested in doing a little more arithmetic, you can use a formula reported by noted researchers Cormillot and Fuchs. It takes steps, so I've given you a worksheet.

Step 1. Determine a hypothetical ideal weight based on the assumption that a woman who is 5 feet tall should weigh about 100 pounds, with 5 pounds added for every inch over 5 feet. (Subtract 5 pounds per inch for those shorter than 5 feet.) If you're 5 feet 6 inches tall, your theoretical ideal weight is 130 pounds.

However, and this is very important, the word *ideal* suggests that this as a goal weight is the exception rather than the rule. For most women, shooting for this value is unreasonable, because it's too low. Most won't have an absolutely ideal history! Rather, there are likely to be several factors which suggest that a weight greater than this ideal prediction is much more reasonable. Do this calculation simply because it is the first step in using the formula to estimate a much more reasonable healthy weight.

Your estimation: Your height = _____ feet _____ inches

"Ideal" weight = _____ pounds

Step 2. Now use Cormillot and Fuchs' formula:

Target weight = Ideal weight + ((age + # yrs overweight) x .22) + (max wt ever/10) - 4.4 (Whew! I hope you like algebra!)

Here are the calculations for Maggie's estimated target weight as an example, so you can see how the numbers work:

height = 5'6"

ideal weight = 100 + (6 x 5) = 130 pounds

age = 38

yrs overweight = 20

max wt ever = 160

Target wt = $130 + ((38 + 20) \times .22) + (160/10) - 4.4$

= 154 pounds

"Wow," exclaimed Maggie, "this value is 15 pounds more than the one I got when I used the lowest weight I had maintained for a year! Shouldn't they be closer to being the same thing?"

"Not at all," I told her. "It simply confirms that there a lot of things to be considered when attempting to predict a healthy weight range. Keep in mind that this formula is simply a statistical prediction. It just gives us an estimation.

"Using the two methods together, let's just say that a reasonable estimate for your healthy weight is somewhere between 140 and 154 pounds. That's pretty close to what Dr. Koop recommends with his 'losing about 10% or more' recommendation."

Here's a worksheet for *you*:

Height = _____

a) ideal weight = _____

b) age = _____

c) # of years overweight = _____

d) max weight ever = _____

Now insert the values (*a, b, c,* and *d*) into the following formula:

$$\text{Target wt} = a\underline{\quad} + ((b\underline{\quad} + c\underline{\quad}) \times .22) + (d\underline{\quad} /10) - 4.4 = \underline{\quad} \text{ pounds}$$

For many women, especially those who've been in the weight loss game for several years, using this weight with the lowest weight you've maintained for a year, like we did with Maggie, may offer a pretty reasonable range.

Body Composition and Percent Body Fat

The scale doesn't tell the whole story. When you step on a scale, the number of pounds displayed doesn't really tell you if it's a healthy weight or not. What appears to be more important from a health point of view is how many of those pounds are fat and how many are everything else (muscle, bones, blood, etc.).

This differentiation is referred to as your body composition. The number of pounds of fat relative to your total weight is called your percent body fat. The rest is usually referred to by exercise physiologists as fat-free mass, or lean body mass. In simpler terms, it's just the percentage of your weight that's not fat. The important thing is that healthy weight is probably more related to percent body fat than it is simply to your total weight.

The most recent research findings suggest that health risks begin to significantly increase if a woman's percentage of body fat goes above somewhere between 26-30%. For men, the health risks become significant above around 19-24%.

The Methods

"Great," you think, *"I'll just do a body composition measurement so I can see if I'm in my healthy weight range."*

The problem is that it's not easy to get an accurate, reliable and repeatable estimation of your percentage of body fat. It takes skill and a lot of practice in using accepted techniques. (In fact, there's even some question about the accuracy of the original scientific research which gave us all the equations we now use to estimate percentage of body fat!)

Just for your information, whenever I use percent body fat estimates for a client, I'm much more interested in being precise with each measurement (so I can determine changes over time) than in focusing on the actual estimate for percentage of body fat.

In recent years, a number of devices have been offered to the public which purport to give you a "quick and easy" reading for your percent body fat. In my opinion, if it's a quick and easy measurement, it's likely to be pretty suspicious.

If you really want to know what your estimated percentage of body fat is, you need to contact a skilled professional. The exercise science or human performance department at a local college or university can probably help you with the most typical research method, called underwater weighing. It's not much fun and it takes about 20 minutes just to do the weighing. But you can do it if you want to!

Underwater weighing has been used by scientists to develop other estimation methods which are quicker and easier, but less accurate. I think that the two most dependable methods used in health clubs and by personal fitness instructors are the ones using skinfold calipers (which measure the thickness of a fold of skin at various sites on your body) or circumference measurements.

I'm not going to go into any detail here, nor am I going to give you charts and formulas for these techniques, because unless you've practiced them a lot, you won't get good results! Who can do them? Here are some suggestions.

- Master members of IDEA, the international association of fitness professionals, have been certified either by the American Council on Exercise (ACE) or the American College of Sports Medicine (ACSM), or they have a college degree in a fitness-related field. Many of these individuals have the necessary skills.

- Fitness instructors and personal fitness trainers certified by ACE or ACSM should also be able to estimate your percentage body fat. Likewise, many registered dietitians have been trained in these techniques.

Do you have to have your percentage of body fat taken? No. It's just another option you have for getting an estimate of your healthy weight range. Is it the best? Not necessarily. In fact, it's probably not as good as the others I've mentioned unless a qualified professional does the measuring!

Height/Weight Charts

Over the years, the height and weight charts based on those initially developed by Metropolitan Life Insurance Company have been used as the standard reference for desirable weights for men and women between the ages of 25 and 59, relative to an individual's height and a never-well-defined "frame size." The charts were developed by statisticians based on the lowest incidence of death (mortality) in their pile of data. The cause of death or health status prior to death were not considered.

Hmm?

Not surprisingly, many experts have long questioned the practical reality of the charts for many people because they don't account for differences in genetic factors, race, age and what you've done for the last 25 years. More importantly, they don't account for the issue of body composition just discussed.

I heartily agree with this opinion! I think there are almost always more reasonable ways to estimate your healthy weight range than using a standard height/weight chart.

So, while the standard chart may be used if you apply for life insurance, the weight range may be totally unrealistic for you!

I continue to feel that height/weight charts provide a rough estimate, at best, for an individual's healthy weight range.

Your Choice

If, like Maggie, you want to at least have some idea of your healthy weight, you now have several different ways you can use to get an estimation. Regardless of which method you might select, remember:

- They are all just estimates. You might be in your healthy range right now!

- Focus on taking care of yourself today, not achieving some future weight goal.

- There's no rush! Most research tells us that maximum *effective* weight loss is about one pound a week.

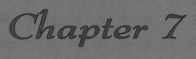

Chapter 7

Managing the Stresses of Everyday Living

This isn't a stress management book. Experts far more qualified than I have written exhaustive texts covering the myriad issues involved in both the psychological and physical aspects of our response to stressful situations. I've included some suggestions in the resources section for those who may be interested in further reading in this area.

But because stress is frequently an issue in real-life weight management, I do want to point out some of the important discoveries regarding the relationship between stress and weight management, as well as some easy—but effective—ways to reduce the potentially negative effects of the stresses of daily living.

This Stress-Overeating Connection

"Maggie," I asked, "You told me that you feel 'stressed-out' more than you'd like to. What does that mean?"

"Well, I guess it's all the stuff that happens to us everyday. Getting kids ready for school, going to work, paying bills, keeping the boss happy. You know, relationships and all that. Never feeling like I have enough time to do all the stuff I'd like to. Eating things I know I shouldn't, at least not as much as I do. And not eating enough of what I know I should. Plus not exercising. I think it all adds up to stress."

I told her that I used to think the same thing—that it was actual events that constituted the stress. That stress was basically bad. That "stress management" meant getting rid of stressful situations.

Turns out that's not it at all. Stress isn't the event itself. Stress is really how we respond to the events of daily living. Stress is unavoidable. And stress can be either good or bad. Good stress? That concept really made me curious!

Research tells us that stress is the response to events that are physical (an injury), chemical (too much caffeine), or emotional (a "bad" day). The response often occurs in all three realms. And it can certainly lead to increased tension.

About 30 years ago, Hans Selye developed his model of the stress response theory as a three-stage process:

1. Alarm

2. Resistance

3. Exhaustion

First, there's **alarm**, or your immediate recognition of the stressful event, often referred to as the "fight or flight" response. It's at this stage that your perception of the event is so important.

If you perceive the event as threatening (which it certainly can be), it can easily lead to emotions of fear, anxiety and/or anger. As you become emotionally aroused, your body produces more of certain hormones which immediately increase your heart rate, blood pressure and blood sugar level. This is good if you have to fight off the imminent attack of a fearsome predator. But when you don't "fight" immediately, you move into the second of Selye's stages: **resistance**.

This second stage potentially has both psychological and physical consequences because the body is resisting the alarm:

Psychological	Physical
lingering anger	headaches
frustration	muscle aches
resentment	digestive problems
distrust/suspicion	increased blood pressure
Depression	*Hunger*

Do you see how reasonable it is for this resistance to make you feel like you're under constant pressure? And look at the last potential consequence in each category! If the alarm phase progresses to the resistance phase, there is a greatly increased chance that you'll be physically and psychologically propelled to overeat! Recent research clearly suggests that this response is directly related to binge eating, or periodically eating a lot of high-calorie foods.

Psychologically, many of us eat when we're depressed. Eating makes us feel better. In fact, there's good evidence to suggest that foods high in simple sugars which women generally binge on increase the production of a chemical in the brain that relieves mental "tension."

Compounding this is the physical reality that the big increase in blood sugar during the alarm phase can make your pancreas produce enough insulin to subsequently drop the blood sugar below "normal," triggering a craving for something sweet. And feeling guilty afterwards only sustains the negative feelings.

Can you relate to this process? If it persists over time, it leads to Selye's third stage: **exhaustion**. By this he's referring to the "exhaustion" of systems in your body—the cardiovascular system, the immune system, etc. This is the stage where there is a big increase in the risk of long-term health problems like high blood pressure, over consumption of calories leading to obesity, chronic depression and so on.

It's hard to escape the "alarm" phase—because we all know those situations are out there! But wouldn't it be great if there was an option to the resistance and exhaustion phases?

Fortunately, there is!

Choosing to Beat Stress

Without the immediate need to "fight," we have the option of perceiving the event as **challenging** rather than threatening. In this way, we can transform the circumstances into a positive stress rather than a negative stress. We can choose to deal with a situation in a calm manner, with conviction and determination.

If it's an injury, let it heal; too much caffeine, cut back; a "bad" day at the office, develop strategies to deal differently with the events of the day.

Which path do you want to follow?

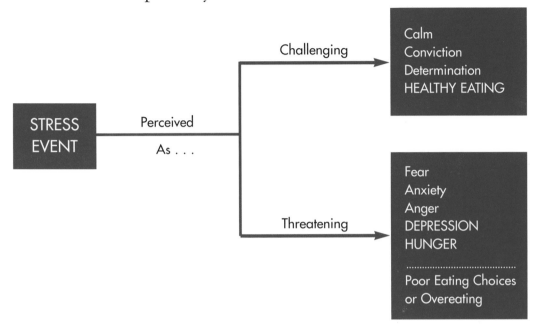

All the things you've decided to do with regard to feeling good about who you are right now will help you immensely in developing stress management skills, the skills to follow the path which enables you to respond to events as representing a positive (challenge), rather than a negative (threat).

As we discussed earlier, it is so easy for us to forget that we all have choices. In fact, it is by recognizing that we have a choice that we empower ourselves to take charge of our health.

And as is true for most everything, different techniques work for different people. And, they do take some practice! There are a number of different ways to develop the skills for taking the it's-a-challenge path.

Practicing the De-Stressing Art

Dr. Herbert Benson, in his book *Your Maximum Mind*, quotes the Dalai Lama, "We human beings have a developed brain and limitless potential. Since even wild animals can gradually be trained with patience, the human mind also can gradually be trained, step by step. With patience, you can come to know this through your own experience."

I will share several methods for handling stress, but there are far more than I'll mention here. The most important thing is that you explore a way (or ways) that works for *you*.

Dr. Benson's Relaxation Response

Developed by Dr. Benson and based on his research into Transcendental Meditation, this method involves four interactive elements for being able to achieve a relaxing effect. You can apply them in a private space in your home or, if you practice, even for brief periods in the midst of the cacophony of life!

To begin with, set aside 15-30 minutes in a quiet place where you can practice this technique.

1. **Use a mental focus.** Repeat a word, a sound, an image, whatever, that you continually bring into focus in your mind, with your eyes closed. This focus must bring about a calming effect. You pick it.

2. **Try a passive attitude.** Disregard the distractions that will undoubtedly come into your mind for whatever period of time—a few moments to several minutes. Allow distracting thoughts to passively "pass through" you rather than engage

your focus. Bring your concentration back to the mental focus you've selected.

3. **Relax your muscles.** This means that you have to be in a comfortable position, sitting or lying down. You can do the relaxation response when you're at your desk by just taking a short break. Or you can do it in the morning, or when you get home after work, for 30 minutes. In any situation it can help you turn the alarm response away from resistance to one of positive challenge.

4. **Make use of a quiet environment.** This might require that you remove yourself from your immediate space, or just "tune it out." That takes practice. Ideally, find a space you have just to yourself for whatever period of time. Kids, spouse, boss, coworkers...no one is to intrude on your space for this period of time.

What I really like about Dr. Benson's technique is that it's not a step 1, step 2…process. Picking a mental focus, refocusing on it when distracting thoughts occur, keeping my muscles relaxed, and creating a quiet environment (even if it's just in my head!) all work together, simultaneously.

You might have to be flexible! Especially at the beginning. But, with practice, this uncomplicated process can have amazing results, as thousands of people have discovered.

From Threat to Challenge: 4 Methods

The *University of California, Berkeley Wellness Newsletter* gives four suggestions for developing the skill to move from being threatened to being challenged by the day's events. I will describe these in terms which are easy to apply:

1. **Scanning.** Stop whatever you're doing. Sit up tall in a comfortable posture, shoulders back, head up. Close your eyes and take a quick "scan" around your body. Where do you feel tight? tense? uncomfortable? Take a moment to focus on and relax the muscles in that area.

2. **Imagery.** Stop whatever you're doing. Visualize in your mind a really pleasant scene. Maybe it's a mountain meadow, the beach, a waterfall, a ballet, whatever. Focus on that image for just a few moments. Enjoy it. Put into perspective whatever was making you feel tense just a few moments ago.

3. **Do "the turtle."** Stop whatever you're doing. (Is this beginning to sound familiar?!) Sit up tall in your chair, shoulders back, head up. Now slowly let your head drop forward until your chin touches your chest. Keep your back straight. Now slowly bring your head up and back until it feels like the back of your head is touching the back of your neck. Do this just a few times to put the "stressor" in perspective. Is it really that big of a deal?

4. **Countdown.** Pick some number, like your age, and slowly count down to zero. (This one takes me awhile!) Focus briefly on each year, and bring one pleasant memory of that year into focus. If nothing comes immediately, that's okay. Just progressively count down, allowing your focus on the countdown to replace the response to the situation which brought about some alarm.

The Jacobson Muscle Relaxation Technique

Dr. E. Jacobson, a physiologist/physician doing research about stress management in the 1930s, gave us quite an effective technique for using a focus on muscle contraction/ relaxation in specific body areas to bring about a very relaxing effect.

There are a number of ways to apply the Jacobson technique, since it has undergone many permutations since the '30s! Here's an easy one:

1. Sit comfortably in a chair. Or lie down on the floor in a relaxing posture.

2. Now progress around your body by selectively contracting, then relaxing muscles in sequential areas. Start from one point—for example, your left foot. Concentrate on contracting just the muscles in your left foot. Then make them completely relax. Move on to the muscles in your lower left leg, then upper left leg, trunk, left hand, left forearm, left upper arm, left shoulder, upper back, neck, chest, right shoulder, right upper arm, and so on, until you get to the right foot.

This is just an example. You can do more body regions at once if you want. The key is to focus your attention first on contracting specific muscles, then on relaxing them.

This technique can have an amazing calming effect.

Equal Count on Breathing In and Breathing Out

This one's my favorite for an immediately calming effect. I find regulated breathing to be immensely helpful if I'm starting to feel stressed.

1. Stop whatever you're doing. (Not surprising, huh?)

2. Breathe in while you count slowly to four (or three, or five).

3. Breathe out while you count the exact same number and rhythm as you did when breathing in.

4. Do this for at least 4 to 5 complete sets.

Find What Works for You

There are a number of other methods you might want to try to help you develop the skills you'll need to turn the stressful events of daily living into positive challenges. Yoga, meditation (Deepak Chopra, MD, recommends that you find a good teacher if you want to learn to use meditation effectively. It's hard to learn it from a book.), biofeedback, visualization, deep breathing, and stretching (see Chapter 11) are all recommended as potentially effective ways for making stress a positive, creative life experience.

I've given you several references in the Resources section if you want more specific information on many of these methods.

Real-Life Stress Prevention

Here are a few other suggestions for how to help reduce the negative stress potential of daily events:

Low-Stress Work Environment

1. Don't bite off more than you can chew. Be able to say, "No, I can't do this right now."

2. Build an effective relationship with your boss.

3. Take time, 2-3 minutes, to relax when you start to feel uptight.

4. Write down your worrisome problems, and your ideas for solutions. Discuss them with your peers and superiors as you feel is appropriate. Don't just keep them to yourself.

5. Reduce unnecessary noise in your work area.

6. Deal with problems ASAP. Don't wait until later.

General

1. Notice when you get angry, irritated or impatient. Write down why you think you are feeling this way. Is there a different way you can respond? Or can you get yourself out of the situation?

2. Try to find the humor in the situation.

3. Spend a minimum of 20 minutes each day in planned relaxation.

4. Watch less violence and highly competitive events on late night TV.

5. Take the time to be neighborly.

6. Set aside time for regular household "conferences" to air disputes and aggravations.

7. Set realistic (but challenging) personal and professional goals.

8. Write down your priorities, then live them—don't wait until later.

9. Talk more slowly and less emphatically in your conversations with others.

10. Take time to really listen to those who are speaking with you. Then construct your response.

11. Make yourself fidget less! Try the breathing trick.

12. Rely on your spiritual beliefs to assist you in keeping perspective.

13. Remember to make the distinction between circumstances within and outside of your control.

14. Never forget that you have a choice in how you respond to events, and try to monitor your responses to ensure that you do not slip into overreacting (e.g., experiencing extreme anger and frustration over a flat tire).

15. *Keep physically fit and eat a sensible diet!* There is no longer any doubt that a lifestyle which incorporates regular physical activity and a sensible diet has a very positive effect on helping you respond well to the stresses of daily living.

This is Your Page to Write Down Your Priorities.

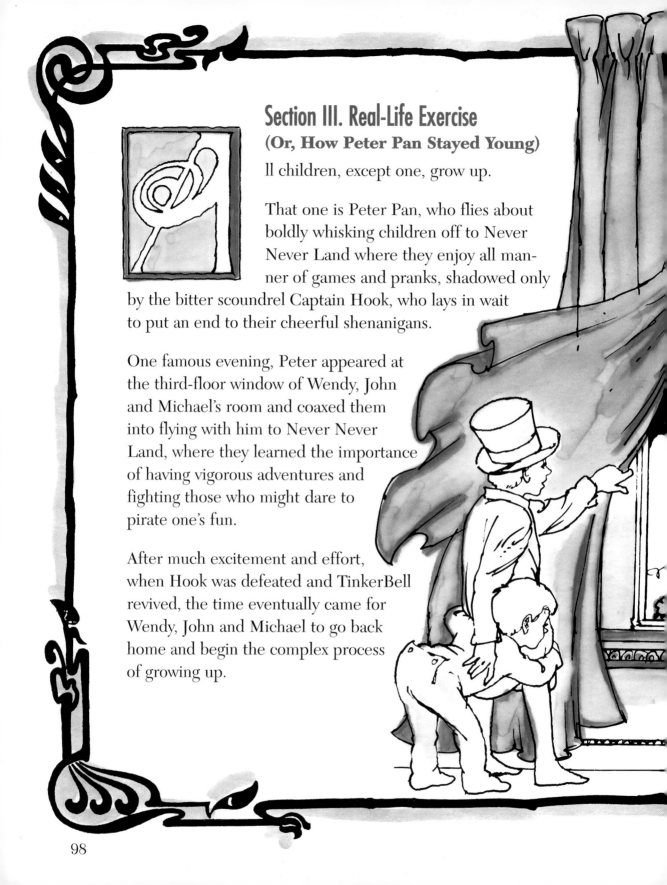

Section III. Real-Life Exercise
(Or, How Peter Pan Stayed Young)

ll children, except one, grow up.

That one is Peter Pan, who flies about boldly whisking children off to Never Never Land where they enjoy all manner of games and pranks, shadowed only by the bitter scoundrel Captain Hook, who lays in wait to put an end to their cheerful shenanigans.

One famous evening, Peter appeared at the third-floor window of Wendy, John and Michael's room and coaxed them into flying with him to Never Never Land, where they learned the importance of having vigorous adventures and fighting those who might dare to pirate one's fun.

After much excitement and effort, when Hook was defeated and TinkerBell revived, the time eventually came for Wendy, John and Michael to go back home and begin the complex process of growing up.

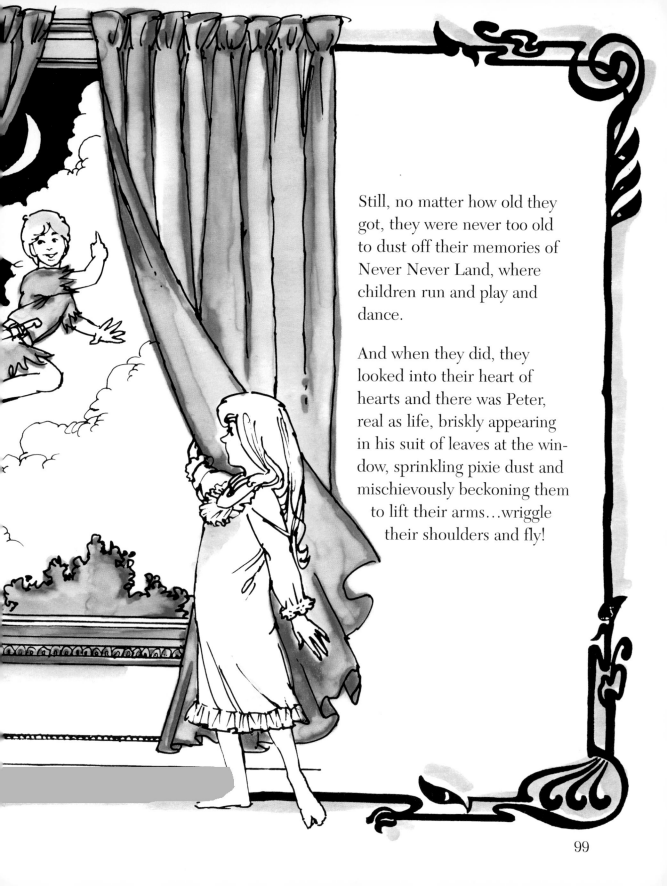

Still, no matter how old they got, they were never too old to dust off their memories of Never Never Land, where children run and play and dance.

And when they did, they looked into their heart of hearts and there was Peter, real as life, briskly appearing in his suit of leaves at the window, sprinkling pixie dust and mischievously beckoning them to lift their arms...wriggle their shoulders and fly!

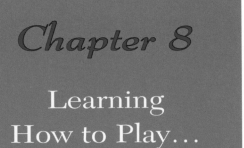

Chapter 8

Learning How to Play... Again

I s exercise a never never land for you? Something you distantly remember from childhood (or at least a few years back)? Your memories may be positive (the fun you had biking around the neighborhood pretending to be flying, or playing basketball in college) or negative (how you hated gym class, and your teacher reminded you of Captain Hook!).

Maybe your closest connection to exercise is someone similar to Peter Pan's little-known stepbrother, Charlie Pan. He's been in an ultimate quest for fitness as long as he can remember, constantly trying to be in better shape than his highly trained, flighty brother. If Peter goes one mile, Charlie thinks he has to go two. If Peter hikes three miles, Charlie has to hike four. If Peter exercises for 30 minutes, Charlie has to work out for an hour.

Like Charlie, your friend probably gets injured a lot. And he doesn't really enjoy his efforts. For Charlie, exercise isn't a way to help manage the stresses in his life. In fact, it adds to his stress levels. He thinks if he misses a day of exercise, he'll lose everything he's gained.

Charlie should pay more attention to his brother's approach! I imagine Peter looking at activity and exercise as parts of enjoying and appreciating life. He sees his body as an amazing machine, which has an immense capacity to move, dance and even "fly!"

How do *you* look at exercise and activity? Drudgery, painful, a hassle, a necessary evil, even punishment? Are you a Captain Hook when it comes to active fun? Or are you a Peter Pan, looking for adventure and reveling in the joy of moving and challenging your body?

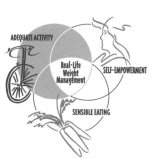

Yes, there is a reason Peter Pan will stay young, active, exuberant (and lean) long after Captain Hook has disappeared from the scene!

The Magic of Real-Life Exercise

If there is any real magic in the weight loss equation, it is probably exercise. Old-style weight management methods either trivialized the role of activity or promoted exercise as a kind of temporary "diet" in itself (for the next six weeks, run six miles a day and go to four aerobic classes a week, etc.).

Today we know from research that one of the few proven predictors of weight maintenance success is regular activity. Perhaps even more importantly, we know that regular activity significantly reduces a long list of health risks, ranging from cardiovascular disease and hypertension to breast cancer.

There are few nicer things you can do for yourself, your body and your future than to become a regular exerciser. Why, then, you might ask, is sticking to an activity program so difficult for so many people? Researchers aren't sure. Once again, the bottom line is that behavior change is rarely easy.

Many experts believe that one reason for the activity-shy trend may be that, just as we have turned healthy eating into a rigid, controlling, unrealistic regimen, we have turned activity into an overly complicated, rigidly demanding and ultimately unrealistic regimen.

We have forgotten what children know—that activity is fun. And we have forgotten that exercise is an act of caring and self-respect (values), not work or punishment.

Before we go any farther, let me add that not every moment of every activity is necessarily "fun." Depending on your personal preferences, there are a variety of aspects of activity (as with anything) that you may not enjoy. However, you might be surprised to find how much there really is to enjoy—especially once you get started and begin to feel comfortable with your new activities.

Just as you may decide to get a college degree even though you don't look forward to the exams, or you may decide to have a child even though you don't look forward to late night feedings (or the teen years!), there will be aspects of your activity program that you won't look forward to—but you will come to find that the benefits make it well worth the trouble.

Regardless of the "fun factor" of your activity program, one thing is certain—nearly everyone enjoys the benefits of having a healthy, invigorated body that moves comfortably and confidently. Think back…was there a time in your life when you had this experience? How did it feel? And if you have never experienced the feeling of a healthy, strong, flexible, well-exercised body—don't be surprised to find that you love it!

What I'm going to do in these next chapters is give you some key fundamentals of exercise which you probably did not learn in physical education classes and you probably aren't familiar with unless you've worked as a fitness professional or with a personal trainer. These fundamentals are not difficult or too scientific to make any sense, but they are key to making your exercise efforts pay off in the best way possible.

I am also going to give you simple, inexpensive options that will allow you to design your own program. Effective fitness takes a little knowledge, but it does not have to be complicated!

Tuning Up

Maggie and I were talking about her experiences with trying to adopt a regular exercise or activity program into her lifestyle. "You know," she told me, "after my very un-fun experience with exercise when I was in college, I've looked at exercise mostly as a punishment. Exercise has never been something that I look forward to. It's something I know I should do, but it's like there's always a good reason to put it off until later."

"Not unusual," I tell her. "In fact, your feelings are shared by many people, even those who aren't necessarily looking at exercise as part of a weight management program. But the reality is that exercise is a vital part of a healthy lifestyle.

Like any machine, our bodies run better when we keep them tuned-up. Exercise is a huge part of the tune-up process. Our muscles work better, our skeleton stays stronger, our hearts work more efficiently and we even sleep better if sensible exercise is part of our lifestyle.

"Regular activity is an especially critical component of successful weight management efforts. But it's only going to work if it can become a pleasurable part of your lifestyle, something you *do* look forward to. Something you see as an important part of taking good care of yourself."

Health Versus Fitness

There is a big difference between becoming more active in order to have a positive impact on *health*, and exercising in order to achieve a high level of *fitness*. This difference is totally related to *how hard*, *how long* and *how often* you participate in whatever activity you choose.

Research has clearly shown that just doing some regular activity, whether it's easy walking, gardening, yard work or recreational doubles tennis, will likely reduce your risk of heart disease. In other words, *you don't have to exercise at a vigorous pace to enjoy some of the health benefits of regular exercise*. This is very important, because some people have a tendency to think that you've got to do a lot to make it worthwhile. For some health benefits, this is absolutely not the case. A little bit can make a big difference.

Achieving a high level of *fitness*, on the other hand, takes some work. That only makes sense. You won't reach a high level of cardiovascular fitness just by working in your garden or taking a stroll around the block.

Anyone who is looking at activity as part of a weight management plan needs to understand that the level of effort put into an activity program will have a big impact on the weight management efforts. This is directly related to a term I bet you're at least somewhat familiar with: **calories**.

The Energy Bank

In the purely physical sense, a large part of real-life weight management relates to the number of calories you take in compared with the number of calories you burn. I like to refer to this as your energy bank. For most of us, in very general terms, if the deposits into our account (calories in from our diet) are greater than the withdrawals (calories burned through resting metabolism and daily activities), we'll put on weight, in the form of fat.

Conversely, if withdrawals are greater than deposits, we'll lose weight. This is called a negative energy balance. *Under the right set of circumstances*, the negative energy balance will lead to weight loss primarily from the body's supply of fat.

Keep in mind that there is a great deal of individual difference in factors which influence resting metabolism. And the type of dietary calories, not just the total number, is certainly important. (We'll look at these nutritional issues in the next section.)

The one issue which is pretty straightforward is the number of calories associated with your activity lifestyle. Many people, like Maggie when she was younger, apply the principles of the energy bank in an ineffective and unhealthy manner.

If you simply restrict eating—decrease the deposits—so calories out are greater than calories in even with little activity, you'll have a negative energy balance and, indeed, you will lose weight. But it won't be just from fat. You'll also lose muscle.

You don't want to do that.

And, according to the so-called set point theory, if you just diet, once you go back to a more normal calorie intake, your body's set point will bring you right back to your former weight, or maybe even higher.

Remember when I told you about resting metabolism—calories burned in basic life processes (heart beating, brain thinking, etc.)? Well, you've got to eat adequate amounts of the right kinds of food each day to provide enough energy for these functions to occur in a healthy way.

If you don't eat enough, your body will convert some of your muscle tissue into a form that can be used to provide this energy. For most adult women "enough" is at least 1,200 calories a day. For men, it's at least 1,500 calories.

The point is this: The energy bank is real. It, like most things, works a little differently from person to person. But the profoundly important relationship between eating enough of the right kinds of food and having adequate activity in effective weight management is indisputable.

The *only* way to increase your body's calorie expenditure in any significant, healthy way is to increase your level of activity. Fortunately, when we are well nourished, the body's main energy reserve is body fat. So, if we can effectively burn more calories than we take in, we'll lose fat. And when we reach a healthy weight, burning the same number as we consume will keep us at our healthy weight.

One final comment on this issue. Some people have taken the energy bank concept to extremes, and this behavior has also been associated with eating disorders. Maggie even tried it: thinking that if she exercised a lot and didn't eat very much, she would really be able to withdraw more calories than she consumed and lose a lot of weight, fast. But over exercising doesn't work in the long run. It's dangerous. Don't do it!

Your car doesn't run very well unless you give it enough of the right kind of fuel. Neither does your body. But if you do give it enough of the right kind of fuel and keep it tuned up, it'll take you to the top of the mountain (or around the block) without a sputter.

Nothing, Something and Fat Loss

I don't want to bore you with a lot of numbers. Nor do I recommend that you become obsessed with the numbers game of comparing calories in with calories out. Becoming too focused on the numbers can easily take you back to old control problems.

There's a lot of individual differences in the way the energy balance equation works, primarily on the calories out side. In some individual situations, the equation doesn't seem to apply very well. The truth is, there's still a lot we don't understand about all of the factors which impact the calorie out part—except that it's not just about exercise.

But it's often helpful to consider some of the basics, such as the fact that doing something (activity) is better than doing nothing (being sedentary) because you burn more calories that way.

Here's what we think we do know. One pound of fat provides approximately 3,500 calories of energy. Because the body prefers to store its primary energy reserve in the form of fat (not protein or carbohydrate), this means that if you want to lose one pound of fat this week, you're going to have to burn 3,500 more calories than you take in. (I don't want to get too academic, but it's important that you realize that one pound of fat loss doesn't translate to exactly one pound of *weight* loss. It's partly why I encourage you to throw your scale out the window!)

When you lose fat, you also lose a bit of water, and some other things. Plus, when you adopt your regular strength training routine, you'll probably add some muscle. So, even though your scale weight may not be changing, you could easily be losing fat! Pay more attention to things like how your clothes fit, and how you feel.

This is where the old potential for eating problems emerges. *"This is simple,"* thought Maggie. *"I'll just knock 500 calories a day off my diet and in 7 days there's my 3,500 calories. In fact, I'll cut out 1,000 calories a day so I can lose 2 pounds of fat this week!"*

However, as you now realize, if you do that, your body will use some muscle to provide for its basic energy needs. And you are likely to be unable to sustain the activity, so you will soon be back where you started—or worse.

"Okay, so I know adequate activity is important, but it seems like it takes so much longer to lose weight that way than to just quit eating. Why is that?" asks Maggie.

"Basically," I tell her, "it's related to the fact that it's a lot easier to eat 1,000 calories than it is to burn 1,000 calories!

Most of us burn about one calorie every minute just being alive, some of us burn a little more, some a little less. That's just another way of describing resting metabolism." (It's also how we know that we need to eat at least 1,200 calories a day to power those processes: 1 cal/min x 60 min/hr x 24 hours/day = approx. 1,400 cal/day.)

"When you go up stairs or walk around the block or work in your garden, ride your bike or play some tennis, you burn more calories every minute. But when you're not in very good condition, it's difficult to sustain an activity which makes you burn more than about 4-5 calories every minute (a brisk walking pace for most of us).

"So, let's say that you decide that you're going to walk for 40 minutes and you burn 5 calories each minute. During that walk you've burned 200 additional calories. If you do that walk three days this week, that's 600 additional calories. At this rate (and at 3,500 calories per pound of fat) it'll take about 6 weeks to drop a pound. I'm assuming you're not making any dietary changes, at this point.

"If you walk for 60 minutes, 5 days a week, the number of calories burned increases a bunch. Sixty minutes times 5 calories each minute times 5 days means you've now burned an additional 1,500 calories this week. So, it'll take just about 2 weeks, rather than 6, to lose that pound of fat.

"One of the really neat things about the body is that if you continue with regular exercise (the next chapter gives specific guidelines), you tremendously increase your ability to burn calories. But it takes weeks and months of regularity.

"Three months from now it's very possible that you can burn 10 calories every minute during your exercise instead of just

5. So, if you do the same 60 minutes, 5 days a week, you'll be burning an additional 3,000 calories each week. That means that you could potentially lose one pound of fat each week on your way to a healthier weight."

I'm not talking 10 pounds in 10 days, because a sensible, healthy approach to weight management doesn't work that way for most people. I hope you can see why.

You may have read about the celebrities who lost a lot of weight in a reasonably short period of time...and kept it off. Consider this: they were most likely exercising for 3-4 hours each day, 5 or 6 days a week. And if they were reasonable about their pace, ate enough nourishing food and drank plenty of water, they could do that in a healthy way.

Do you have that much time available? If not, just be patient. The Oprahs and the Susan Powters of the world have discovered after unsuccessfully trying the quick fix, starvation diet approaches, that the one best long-term approach is to add as much activity as is reasonable in your situation (and eat enough). The more you can add, the more quickly you can expect to see changes.

In the next three chapters, I'm going to give you some specific suggestions for incorporating three distinctive types of activity into your lifestyle: cardiovascular (aerobic), strength and stretching.

General Guidelines for an Active Lifestyle

Doing some activity is more healthful than doing nothing. But the reality is that if you want to ultimately "burn off" excess body fat, you're going to have to improve your level of fitness. But this isn't bad news. Exercise doesn't need to be of the exhausting, I've-been-run-over-by-a-truck variety in order to be effective in the long run. In fact, that's exactly the *wrong* kind of exercise.

There is a huge difference between the way a competitive athlete must exercise in order to try to win a competition, and the way the rest of us need to exercise to achieve a good level of fitness. The athletes work long and hard, and accept a relatively high risk of injury. We don't need to exercise anywhere near that hard or that often. Unfortunately, many people think that they need to work at the athlete's level.

Exercising for fitness is a much different ball game than exercising for performance. The key to getting fit is getting active: The more active, the more fit. But it doesn't need to hurt, and the risk of injury is usually very low.

Your activity/exercise program is like a triangle. I call it the Exercise Triangle.

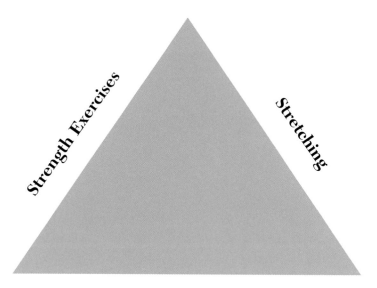

Cardiovascular Activities

The bottom side is cardiovascular (aerobic) activity—that's the next chapter. The triangle's two sides are muscle strengthening exercises and stretching postures—that's two more chapters. They are all important. They all lead to unique benefits. But none of them have to take up all that much time!

Can you give yourself at least five hours each week (that's five hours out of 168 hours—less than 3% of your weekly living time—that you're going to commit to becoming healthier) to becoming more active? Your time commitment can include aerobic, strength and flexibility exercises—that's right, all in five hours a week!

It's one of the best investments you'll ever make. And with the plan you can develop here, it doesn't have to cost you more than a good pair of shoes and some comfortable clothing.

So much for my pitch. I don't have any magic fat-burning schemes. I just want you to be able to burn more calories, get stronger and stay flexible.

As we said, you don't have to follow the workout program of competitive athletes to accomplish the calorie-burning goal which will put you on your way to real-life weight management. But you are going to have to put forth some effort. That's the challenging part: using the positive stress of physical activity to your advantage. You'll be amazed at how much more energy and self-confidence you'll have when you activate your activity plan!

Think of the ingredients of your activity programs as:

- **The type(s)** of activities you're going to do. This is the various kinds of aerobic, strengthening, and flexibility activities and exercises. Fortunately, there's a lot more than one for each side of the activity triangle.

- **The intensity.** This describes how "hard" you work, or your level of effort. I'll give you some easy ways to make sure you're doing your activities hard enough to give you lots of benefits, but not too hard. Remember, "No Pain, No Gain" is not the motto to work by!

- **The duration.** This is simply how long each session should last.

- **The frequency**, or how often you need to do an activity to reap the benefits.

Before we get to the specifics of the Exercise Triangle, let's consider what I suspect is a (the) most crucial aspect of your personal activity plans—staying with them. It's likely that you realize being active is important. You've probably even thought about and tried getting into some kind of regular routine, perhaps several times.

The unfortunate reality is that the majority of those who start a regular program of exercise quit within six months. So, it's not a question of understanding the importance. It may be more a question of creating the lifestyle environment which allows it to continue.

Turn back to Chapter 3 where you considered some of your personal feelings about activity. As you do that, consider the following most common reasons that people give for not staying with a regular exercise routine:

Reason	Potential Solution
1. Medical problems	Consult with a physician and a fitness professional to develop a safe, effective routine. Many conditions do NOT preclude activity and may be helped if you become more active.
2. Last time I tried I got hurt and had to stop.	You may have tried to do too much, too fast. Carefully consider the guidelines in the next 3 chapters so you can progress in a safe and effective manner with little risk of injury.
3. I don't have time.	A. There are 24 hours in a day. Say you sleep for 8-9 and work for 9, that leaves 6-7 hours for everything else. 30-60 minutes of activity for your health seems pretty reasonable!
	B. Use a stroller or a bike seat to take your kid(s) on your walk or ride.
	C. Schedule your regular exercise "appointments" into your daily calendar just like you do business meetings and luncheons.
	D. Put an exercise machine in front of the TV while you watch Peter Jennings on the news.
	E. If your doctor told you to come in for treatment of (you name it) problem, would you tell her that you don't have time?
4. I'm too tired.	If you do it right, it'll probably give you an immediate boost, and more energy in the long run!

Reason – continued	**Potential Solution – continued**
5. I'm too embarrassed.	Don't forget that the people who care about you don't care because of the way you look; they care because of who you are. They'll likely be thrilled that you're taking this step to improve your health.
6. I'm too stressed out.	Look back through Chapter 7. Done sensibly, regular exercise will probably help you deal more effectively with life's daily stresses.
7. I'm just not motivated.	A. Recent studies suggest that using a personal trainer is an excellent way to get going and to stay with your exercise plan. Check the Resources section for more about find a personal trainer.
	B. Find an exercise partner, a fitness friend, a person who will exercise with you. Someone at about your level of fitness is usually best. Schedule regular times so you will need to be there for your fitness friend.
	C. Join a support group made up of people who simply need someone to exercise with. If there isn't one, you can even start one! In the Resources section, you'll find information on how you can start such a group.
	D. Put your exercise apparatus and clothing in conspicuous places. That way it won't be "out of sight, out of mind!"

One final note before we get into specifics about various types of activities: Be sure you get a complete physical examination from your physician before you begin your exercise program. Let her know that you're committed to starting a program, so any medical considerations can be addressed prior to beginning.

Now let's look at the sides of the Exercise Triangle individually.

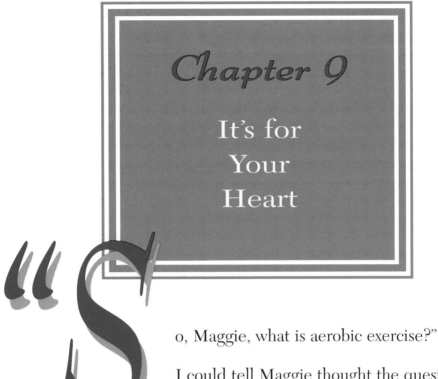

Chapter 9

It's for Your Heart

"So, Maggie, what is aerobic exercise?"

I could tell Maggie thought the question was a little stupid, but she humored me. "Isn't that when you're in a big group of people doing low impact, high impact or step choreography? The class has to be led by a thin, young, energetic instructor. Like the stars on the exercise videos I buy...and hardly ever use. Or on those television fitness shows. Isn't that aerobics?"

"Well, that's what a lot of people seem to think. But that's only one kind of so-called 'aerobic' exercise. It will probably surprise you to discover that sitting in your chair watching TV is an 'aerobic' activity! But you're not burning very many calories."

I won't bore you with a bunch of biochemistry about the real meaning of the words *aerobic* and *anaerobic*. Or how your muscles burn fatty acids (fat) and glucose (sugar). Or the incredible misuse and misrepresentation of the phrase *fat-burning* in trying to sell products and programs.

Understanding the why isn't our purpose here. What I hope you can understand and *apply* is the how. In the annals of consumer marketing for weight management programs and products, the fat-burning phrase will undoubtedly go down as the most widely used, unscientifically applied attempt to beguile unsuspecting customers into believing that there's some magic or uniquely powerful way to burn more fat!

"The best fat-burning machine you'll ever have!"

"This bar will actually help you 'burn fat faster'!"

"Take this pill before/during/after (take your pick!) meals to increase your fat-burning potential."

"... scientific proof that this 'product' will actually help you burn more fat while you sleep!"

"Wear this belt around your waist while you exercise and see your waist size shrink 3 inches in an hour!" (All from water loss. But they forgot to tell you that.)

While they all were lured into trying the too-good-to-be-true pitches, Oprah Winfrey, Susan Powter and Richard Simmons all now tell you that the "secret" to effective weight management is getting as active as you can and eating a sensible diet! Don't be fooled by the outrageous claims you continue to be assaulted with!

The key to losing excess body fat, and keeping it off for the rest of your life, is burning *more calories through activity than you take in from a nourishing, adequate-calorie diet.*

Here are the basics about aerobic exercise. *Aerobic* simply means "with oxygen." The key to effective aerobic exercise is to use large muscles in activities where the heart can supply them with enough oxygen. Let's look at aerobic exercise in terms of type, intensity, duration and frequency.

Type of Exercise

Basically, any activity that makes you keep moving your legs—or arms, if moving the legs is not an option—in a rhythmic, continuous fashion is the easiest way to gain aerobic benefits. You can also burn more calories in a shorter time, in general, with these types of activities. Walking is often suggested as a great way to burn calories and improve your cardiovascular fitness. And it is. But it's certainly not the only way. And, the reality is that unless you're a race-walker or you walk up steep hills, you probably won't burn as many calories each minute as with many other types of activities. However, it is a great way to start, costs no more than a good pair of walking shoes, and can be done almost anywhere.

It's also easier to find a partner to go with you to walk than to engage in some other types of aerobic activities. As a reminder regarding an exercise partner, try to find someone who's at about your level of aerobic fitness. Someone who's more fit might encourage you to go at too great an intensity for your current level. Someone who's less fit will probably keep you from gaining the most from your time spent. And, like most of us, you are probably fitting your activities into an already busy schedule!

What about other activities that can have good aerobic benefits? Cycling, cross-country skiing, skating, in-line skating, stair climbing, aerobics classes, swimming, rowing...the list goes on. Working arms and legs together gets a lot of muscles going, but contrary to the claims of certain equipment manufacturers, you are not guaranteed to burn more calories every minute using their machine than if you just use your legs. I assure you that an elite marathon runner burns a lot more calories each minute during a race than when she straps on her cross-country skis and goes for a leisurely cruise through the woods!

Activities like tennis, racquetball, volleyball and so forth must be played at an aggressive pace to yield the same aerobic benefits as rhythmic, continuous activities. If you play at the level of world class tennis, racquetball, or two-person beach volleyball players, you're definitely burning lots of calories! However, most of us don't play at that level.

These are, however, great activities and can certainly be a part of your lifestyle activity plan. If weight loss is a goal, you just have to accept the reality that it may take a bit longer to get there than if you can also include some of the more rhythmic, continuous kinds of exercise. But we're talking about a lifestyle plan, and besides, what's the rush? Right? If these are the things you'll do, then these are the ones for you.

How about golf and bowling? Great fun! But what do you think about the aerobic challenge? If you briskly walk the 18-hole course carrying your bag, yes. If you ride in a cart, not much. And if you drink sodas or beer while in the cart...!

Getting Started

"Maggie, as with all this stuff, you have to choose which

type of activity you'll do. Something is better than nothing. But in all honesty, some activities are better at burning calories than others. You decide which one(s) you're most likely to stick with. You're much more likely to stay with the ones you enjoy.

"One final word here, since we're talking about something which is becoming part of your lifestyle, don't get too hung up on the enjoyment part, especially right now. You might tell me you don't like any of these. None of them sounds 'fun.' I just want you to know that there are lots of days when I can easily talk myself out of an activity session beforehand—for a million different reasons.

"But I'll tell you this. I can't remember a time when I didn't feel better afterwards. Not just physically, but mentally. It feels good to make a decision to include activity in your lifestyle and then do it. It's a great way to feel good about yourself.

"So, if you're under the impression that you're always going to like the thought that now's the time to work out, or that you have to, I don't agree. You're doing this—becoming more active—because it's part of taking care of yourself, of feeling good about who you are today. And I know that if I do that session that I just tried to talk myself out of, I always feel good about doing it when I'm done."

"Yeah," Maggie replied. "A lot of the time it made me feel good about myself when I went to my aerobics class or rode the bike. And I do think that maybe getting back into those would be nice, plus walking. But there were times when I didn't feel very good after a session. I was exhausted, and sometimes my legs hurt, not just then, but the next day."

"That doesn't surprise me, from what you've told me about the way you approached your exercise habit," I replied. "Keep in mind that type, intensity, duration and frequency all work together, like a team. I suspect that your discomfort came from the fact that you worked too hard, perhaps too long, and maybe even too often. Especially at the beginning.

"One of the most amazing things about our bodies is how dramatically they can improve their ability to be active, particularly when you haven't been active for awhile. While I fully acknowledge that it's going to take a lot of commitment to stay with your plan for the first six months, try to make yourself do it. Your habit now is not to be active—you've got to make a new habit.

"The vast majority of people who begin exercise programs drop out within the first six months. If you can stay with it for that long, it is very likely that exercise will become a part of your lifestyle.

"I don't guarantee many things! But I will guarantee (almost!) that if you can stay with your plan for that long you will look forward to your sessions much more often than you do now. I don't always look forward to mine, but I do most of the time!

"Now, let's talk about how hard—the intensity—you should do your walking, aerobics, and cycling."

Intensity—How Hard

There are several different ways to monitor how hard you are working. Most of what you've read and heard has probably suggested that you keep your heart rate between a lower and a higher value (your target heart rate range) that you select from a chart based on your age.

Target Heart Rate Range Chart

Age	60%		85%	
	Monitor Beats/Min	Pulse Beats/10 Sec	Monitor Beats/Min	Pulse Beats/10 Sec
20	120	20	170	28
25	117	20	166	28
30	114	19	162	27
35	111	19	157	26
40	108	18	153	26
45	105	18	149	25
50	102	17	145	24
55	99	17	140	23
60	96	16	136	23

If you're just beginning you should stay toward the lower value in your training range. As you get more fit you can probably work more comfortably toward the higher value. In all situations pay attention to your breathing (the"Talk Test"). Use the heart rate range as a reference.

If you are using a heart rate monitor, the beats/minute values are what you should use. If you're checking a pulse at your wrist, use the beats/10 second values. Place the pads of your first two fingers gently on the outside of your wrist just below the thumb to locate your pulse. Then count the number of beats in a 10-second period.

I've put together a chart in this chapter that gives you this heart rate range from 60-85% of your maximum predicted heart rate. Using a chart like this works for lots of people. But, in truth, I don't recommend that you use a target heart rate as the only way you monitor your pace unless you do a graded exercise test, administered by your physician or other qualified professional.

During this test, your heart rate must be monitored. That's the only way to accurately determine your target zone. (I recommend that you have this done if you're over 40 and haven't been exercising for awhile.)

The problem with the chart is that your maximum heart rate is predicted by subtracting your age from 220. Maggie's predicted maximum heart rate is 220 - 38 = 182 beats/minute. The reality is that her true maximum heart rate may be as many as 10 to 15 beats/minute higher or lower than her predicted value.

On the chart I've given the ranges based on five-year age increments, but understand that the error in prediction is as true for you as it is for Maggie.

If you don't have a graded exercise test, and I know many of you won't, I still want you to become more active. So use the target heart rate as a general reference. (I must also tell you that a lot of people do not accurately measure their pulse at the wrist or at the neck. If you really want to know your heart rate during exercise, I recommend that you buy a monitor. Choose one which includes a transmitter that you strap across your chest, which sends your heart rate to a receiver you wear like a watch. I've given you a reference in the Resources section if you want one.)

Pay as much or more attention to how you feel during your exercise session as you do to what your heart rate is. Here are three excellent ways to monitor your pace:

1. **Use the "talk test."** If you're exercising at a good pace, of course you'll be breathing more deeply and more rapidly than when sitting in a chair. But if you are beginning to struggle to get enough air, it's time for you to slow down. The talk test: If you can sing a whole song without taking a breath, you're not working hard enough, but if you can't string 3-4 words together comfortably, you're working too hard. Slow down, to a pace which allows you to comfortably talk and exercise at the same time.

2. **"Burning muscles."** By-products of muscle effort, such as lactic acid, can build up in exercising muscles. If you're starting to work at a pace beyond your aerobic level, this buildup occurs very quickly. And these byproducts make your muscles feel uncomfortable or achy (i.e., you "feel the burn"). For aerobic fitness exercise you don't want this to happen. So if the muscles you're using (like your thighs if you're walking) start to "burn" during your walk, slow down to a pace at which they do not burn. Then continue at that pace.

3. **"How long can I keep up this pace?"** One of the great things about exercise is that it can really teach you to "listen" to your body. And in the process, it can be a great stress management tool! Exercise takes your mind away from those potentially negative stressful events and focuses you on what you're doing right now. I encourage you to have a little conversation with yourself while you're exercising. Ask yourself, "How long can I keep up this pace?" If the answer is, "I could do this all day long," you might want to pick up your pace a bit!

On the other hand, if the answer is, "Whew! another 5 minutes at this pace and I'm done!" you should slow down. Work at a pace where the answer is something like, "Yes, I'm working, but I'm comfortable. I can keep this up for 20 or 30 more minutes."

As you become more fit, you'll find that a pace which 2 or 3 months ago left you breathless, with "burning" muscles, is now easy to keep up. If you're using your heart rate to monitor, you'll discover that a pace which used to easily take you into your zone is not enough. In other words you can work harder and harder and still be in your aerobic exercise zone!

And that means you'll be burning more and more calories every minute.

You can go from burning at most 4-5 calories a minute to—6 months from now—burning 10-12 or more calories per minute. And you'll be just as comfortable, maybe more, than when you started.

It all depends on whether you stick with your plan.

Interval Exercise

Endurance athletes have used interval training for years because it has such a powerful effect on their performance training. I encourage you to use *fitness intervals*, not the performance intervals used by competitive athletes. Performance intervals take you to exhaustion (remember Bill?) Fitness intervals make you work but not uncomfortably. Here's what a fitness interval workout might look like:

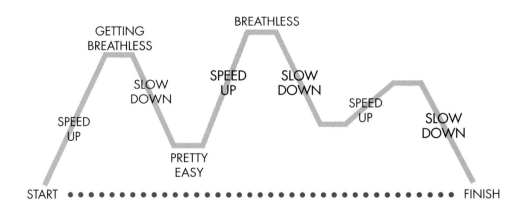

Use the same techniques (breathing, feelings in muscles, ability to maintain pace) to monitor your pace. Essentially, all you do is speed up and slow down during your exercise session, rather than working at a constant pace. Several potential advantages are:

- it breaks up the session into several small intervals

- it allows your muscles some recovery even while you're exercising

- it enables you to burn more calories during your workout

- it leaves you still feeling good, not exhausted at the end of your workout

- it helps you improve your level of fitness more rapidly

You can do intervals with any kind of aerobic activity—walking, cycling, running, swimming…. Unlike performance intervals, fitness intervals are yours to play with—no set time for speed up and slow down. The Scandinavians calls this "speed play" (fartlek training). Play during your exercise session. Sometimes speed up quickly, take awhile to slow down. Next interval, slowly speed up until you start to become breathless (or your heart rate hits the top value, or your muscles start to burn a little).

You'll probably discover that the harder part of interval exercise is the slowing down, not the speeding up part!

Duration—How Long

How long should each session last? The longer, the better (within reason!). Ten minutes is better than five. Fifteen is better than ten. The key is to work long enough, at the right pace, so that you will burn enough calories to count in your energy bank.

Recent research tells us that you can do three 5-minute sessions in a day and get the same benefits as in one 15-minute session. That's great news!

If you can go for a brisk 30-minute walk in the morning and a brisk 30-minute walk in the evening, that'll give you the same health and calorie-burning benefits as one 60-minute session.

Now, let's be real for a second. True, doing something is better than doing nothing. Five minutes of exercise is better than no minutes of exercise. But if you want to lose excess fat, I encourage you to plan at least 20-30 minutes per session.

If you're just starting, remember that you'll probably be able to burn, at the appropriate intensity, about five calories per minute. So, each session will take 100-150 calories out of your energy reserve.

If this is your duration, it'll obviously take longer to create that negative 3,500-calorie balance to lose a pound of fat (remember this is not necessarily what you see on the scale). If you can go for a total of 60 minutes, that bumps your withdrawal up to 300 calories. You decide. Just be realistic in your expectations.

And remember that as your fitness level improves, you're

going to be able to burn 200-300 calories or more during a 20-30 minute session. Be patient, but persistent.

Frequency—How Often

How often is much the same as how long. It depends on your schedule. I encourage everyone to take at least one day a week for complete rest and relaxation. Your body—and your mind—needs it. If Maggie can walk, cycle and do aerobics five or six days a week, she'll burn more calories than if she only does them three days a week. If she goes for 20 minutes, six days a week, that's the same as 40 minutes, three days a week.

Let's look at the numbers:

- Five calories a minute, 60 minutes a day, 6 days a week = 1,800 calories a week. No changes in diet. That's about a pound of fat loss every two weeks.

- Five calories a minute, 20 minutes a day, 3 days a week = 300 calories a week. It'll take a lot longer to lose a pound of fat—2 to 3 months. (Again, if that's the only change in lifestyle.)

I'm telling you all this because it's just the reality of the situation. The longer, the harder (using the guidelines for intensity), and the more often you can exercise, the more calories you're going to burn and the more rapidly your fitness will improve. This adds up to the fact that as your level of fitness improves, the rate at which you can lose fat will also increase, dramatically.

I do not tell you this to take you back to "a little exercise isn't worth it" thinking! Don't forget what I said in the beginning: every little bit counts in your health's favor. Fat loss is a nice bonus, but the *big* benefit is a healthier, stronger, more efficient heart.

It all depends on what your goals are. If you just take it day by day, then it really doesn't matter how long you keep working toward a goal. But there's also a lot of motivation potential in seeing results. So, keep it in perspective. Make aerobic exercise a part of your lifestyle.

Does this help you understand why your friend (or maybe even you) who takes a leisurely 20-minute walk around the block two or three times a week probably doesn't experience a lot of body composition changes?

If the goal was weight loss, and this is the exercise program, I will bet that it won't last. Results are slow, expectations aren't met and the resulting thinking says, "This exercise isn't working. Maybe I'll just try another diet."

If you've followed the story of Oprah Winfrey at all, you'll recognize that her effective weight maintenance has occurred since she's been training for and running marathons. That's a lot of calories out of the energy bank every week!

Just as I am not going to ask you to count your dietary calories every day, I'm asking you not to count your exercise calories. I think it causes you to be too focused on the wrong thing. Just get active.

As you become more fit, you can exercise harder (and longer) and you'll certainly burn more calories. If you want more detailed information on calories burned in various activities, see the Resources section.

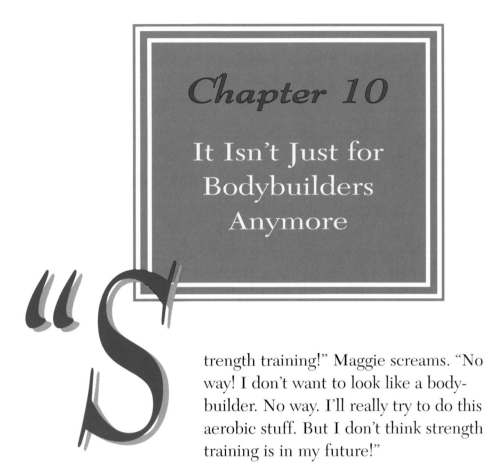

Chapter 10

It Isn't Just for Bodybuilders Anymore

"**S**trength training!" Maggie screams. "No way! I don't want to look like a bodybuilder. No way. I'll really try to do this aerobic stuff. But I don't think strength training is in my future!"

I had to admire Maggie's honesty. And this is a relatively common way to think, especially among people who haven't exercised for awhile. But strength training doesn't necessarily mean making *bigger* muscles; it means making *stronger* muscles. Muscles don't have to get bigger to get stronger. And actually, in most women, muscles won't get much bigger even if you work pretty hard.

Women generally don't have the genetics for that kind of adaptation. But muscles will get a lot stronger. It has to do with changes that happen inside muscle cells, which pack them more full of the stuff that make them strong. A quiver filled with 15 arrows has a lot more firepower than the same quiver with only eight arrows. The quiver's not any bigger; it's just more fully packed.

Some women, just by genetics, naturally have more of a particular hormone (testosterone) than other women do, just like the natural differences that occur between men. But most men have more testosterone than most women. That's a major reason why most men who strength train reasonably hard will get bigger muscles—and why most women, even if they train pretty hard, won't get much bigger muscles. A particular woman with a naturally higher testosterone level who trains hard may get bigger muscles.

However, if you do the strength exercises shown in this book your muscles won't get that much bigger, regardless!

Why Should I Do Strength Exercises?

Many of us who've been in the fitness business for awhile were thrilled when the American College of Sports Medicine (ACSM) included a recommendation for strength exercises in their most recent guidelines. Strength doesn't just have to do with sports performance. It has to do with health.

Keeping your muscles strong (and your joints flexible—next chapter) helps reduce your risk of injury, like when you're doing your aerobic activities, playing with your kids, or going for a week's vacation at the beach or ski area.

Strong muscles help you keep a confident, self-assured posture. As you age, "imbalances" in strength develop between muscles that cause movements at the various joints in your skeleton, like between the muscles on the front of your chest and shoulders, and the muscles in your upper back and the backs of the shoulders. The imbalances are likely a major contributor to the posture problems that many people experience when they get to be 40, and 50, and 60...

One of the best ways to prevent, halt and sometimes even correct these problems is to strengthen the muscles, bringing back a good balance between the opposing muscle groups in your body. Sure, this takes some work. But not nearly as much as you might think.

Remember the five hours a week you said you'd commit to in Chapter 9? After reading that chapter, I hope you'll dedicate three hours to aerobic exercise. If you'll add just 20-30 minutes, twice a week, for strength exercises, you'll get stronger muscles and still have an hour a week left for stretching. That's plenty. (I hope you're thinking, "This can work!")

Perhaps one of the most compelling reasons to include strength exercises, especially for women, is the growing evidence that this type of exercise may be one of the best ways to reduce the risk of osteoporosis as we age. Osteoporosis, often thought of as a woman's problem, occurs in both women and men. But because of hormonal changes that occur after menopause, women typically have a somewhat higher risk. Include strength exercises in your activity plan, and you reduce your risk.

If you're over 50 it's definitely not too late to start! Research suggests that people in their 70s and 80s can make substantial strength gains, even if they haven't exercised for years. While it's too soon to know if osteoporosis can be reversed with strength exercises, it's likely that such activity can halt the progression.

And because we're talking about weight loss, I've saved the

best reason to do strength exercises for last. When you make muscles stronger, they *burn more calories every day*. The exact number is still controversial, but it's likely that for each pound of muscle you make with your strength exercises, you add at least 20-30 calories a day to your resting energy output. That may not sound like much, but 20 times 365 days a year is 7,300 calories.

It certainly adds up.

There are a number of recent studies which clearly suggest that doing both strength and aerobic exercises, and eating a sensible diet, is probably the best way to get to a healthier weight.

Strength Guidelines

The exercises I've given to you in this chapter don't require any equipment. They're designed to get you started on a regular strength routine. I think that once you start to feel the benefits that these exercises give you, many of you will want to explore the realm of strength training with free weights, machines, elastic resistance bands or tubes. You might also want to try some water exercise classes. Not only can they give you a great aerobic workout, but the resistance provided by the water also helps you strengthen your muscles.

I heartily recommend that you get professional guidance from a qualified personal trainer or fitness instructor. There are certainly lots of books, videos and magazines that show you different strength exercises. In fact, I've worked on and helped write several of them. But I have to tell you that it's not easy to learn correct form, posture and technique without someone right there with you. You can, but it's not easy, especially if you've never done it before.

Hiring an IDEA personal trainer who's certified by the American Council on Exercise (ACE), American College of Sports Medicine (ACSM), or the National Strength and Conditioning Association (NSCA) may be a smart move for you. You might only need the trainer to come to your house for a few times, just to show you how to do the exercises safely and effectively.

She or he can tell you all about sets, reps (repetitions), how much weight to use, and when you should increase or decrease the amount of resistance. And, very importantly, a trainer can help you modify an exercise if the one you've seen just isn't comfortable for you.

You may also find that having a personal trainer is just what you need to keep you on track with your plan. The Resources section gives you information on how to locate a qualified personal trainer in your area.

The *Get Real* Strength Guidelines

The eight exercises that follow work most of the major muscle groups. Just a couple of general comments:

- Always breathe when you're doing strength exercises. Breathe out on the hard (effort) part of the movement, and inhale on the easier part (recovery).

- Count two seconds for the effort part, two seconds for the recovery part. You'll hear other breathing rhythm suggestions. There's no real evidence that any particular rhythm is the best. Two for effort, two for recovery works, and it's easy for most beginners to remember.

- Do the exercises with smooth, controlled movements, in both directions. Don't do rapid, jerky movements. If you can't complete one repetition—one effort, one recovery—stop. Don't try to force it.

- If a particular exercise causes pain in a joint, or is just plain uncomfortable, don't do it.

- Since for many of you, these may be the first strength exercises you've done in quite some time (maybe ever!), you can expect a little stiffness and soreness in the muscles the day after you've exercised. It's just a sign they're responding to this positive stress. If you stay with it for a few weeks, this delayed soreness won't occur when you do these exercises.

- Use a mirror if at all possible to check your posture while doing these exercises.

- A repetition (rep) is one complete movement—effort and recovery.

- A set is one series of a given number of reps—for example, one set of 10 reps of a given exercise. When you progress to doing two sets, rest for about a minute between sets.

Try doing the following sequence of eight exercises two or three times a week, for six weeks. It will only take you 20-30 minutes each time. Remember, these exercises will not "bulk you up," they will just give you added strength for your daily activities and help you enjoy the benefits of feeling stronger and more fit! You don't have to do them in any specific order.

You may experience some resistance to doing these, such as telling yourself they're "too hard" or "too boring." Try not to listen! Tell yourself instead that this is a simple, time-efficient way to take care of yourself and have more enjoyable, productive days!

SQUATS

(Strengthens thighs, buttocks, calves)

Stand tall, hands on hips, feet slightly wider than shoulders, toes slightly turned out. Bend your knees, ankles and hips as you inhale and control your movement down toward the floor. Your neck and back should stay lined up; your torso should bend slightly forward at the hip (not in the lower back). Start by just going down until your knees are at about a 45 degree angle (see illustration). Exhale as you straighten your legs and hips, pushing yourself back up to the starting position.

Start with one set of 5-8 repetitions to the 45 degree position. When you can comfortably do two sets of 10-12, move on to one set of 5-8 going down to a right angle at your knees (see illustration). Work up to two sets of 10-15 reps.

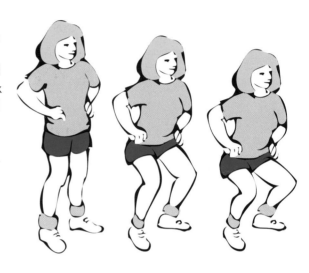

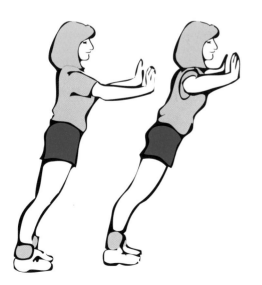

WALL PUSH-UPS

(Strengthens backs of arms, chest, and fronts of shoulders)

Stand with your feet slightly wider than shoulder width, lean forward and put the palms of your hands on a wall, about 6-8 inches wider than your shoulders. Inhale as you bend your elbows and control your movement toward the wall. Keep your head up, back straight, knees just slightly flexed. Now exhale as you push away from the wall, using your chest, arms and shoulders.

Start by doing one set of 5-8 complete repetitions (movements). When you can comfortably do two sets of 10-12 repetitions, with one minute of rest between sets, move to the modified push-up.

137

MODIFIED PUSH-UP

Start with your hands in the same position as for the wall push-up, except place them on the floor. Resting on your knees, keep your neck, back and thighs lined up. Inhale as you bend your elbows, controlling your movement down until your chest nearly touches the floor. Exhale as you push yourself back up to the starting position.

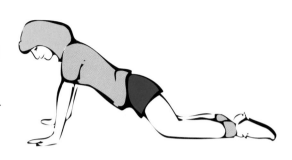

As before, when you can comfortably do two sets of 10-12 reps, move to the full push-up.

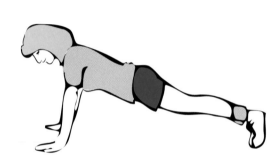

FULL PUSH-UP

Use the same hand position as in the modified, but now your legs are straight, toes on the floor. Maintain good alignment from the neck, through your torso and legs, to your feet. Inhale down, exhale as you push up. Maintain alignment throughout the movement.

Work up to a maintenance level of two sets of 10-15 reps.

BENT-OVER LATERAL RAISE

(Strengthens backs of shoulders, upper back)

Sitting in a chair as shown, rest your chest on your thighs, arms down at your side. Keeping your elbows just slightly bent, exhale as you lift your arms straight out to the side, not back. Inhale as you control your arm movement down.

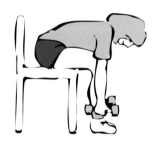

Start with one set of 8-10 reps. Work up to two sets of 10-15 repetitions. When you get to this point, you might want to pick up some three and five pound handweights to keep strengthening these muscles. Use the same guidelines for sets and reps if you do get handweights.

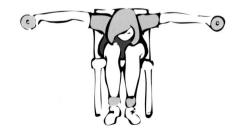

STANDING LUNGE

(Strengthens thighs, hips, calves)

Start by holding onto the back of a chair as shown. Put the foot that is farther away from the chair about 12-15 inches in front of you. Extend the leg that is closer to the chair behind you so you balance on those toes. Inhale as you bend both knees and let your torso drop straight toward the floor, not forward. Your front knee stays over the front foot. Go down until your front knee is at a right angle. Exhale as you press yourself straight up.

Start by doing one set of 5-8 repetitions, repeat to other side. When you can do two sets of 10-15 reps, you can do them with your hands on your hips. It's great for balance.

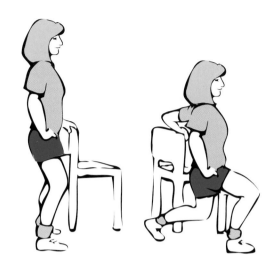

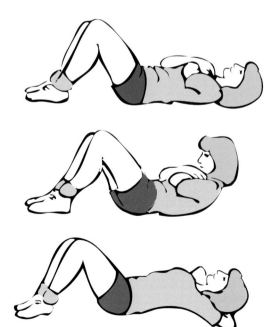

ABDOMINAL CURL-UPS

(Strengthens abdominals)

Start by lying on your back, knees bent, feet flat on the floor, hands crossed on your chest. Exhale as you curl your torso up just until your shoulder blades are off the floor. Inhale as you go back down. Keep your neck straight throughout the movement, up and down.

Start with one set of 5-8 reps. When you can do two sets of 10-15, you can bring your hands behind your head to make it a little harder. But don't pull your head forward as you come up. Instead, press your head back into your hands as you come up. (It takes a little practice!)

REVERSE TRUNK CURLS
(Strengthens abdominals)

This is a difficult exercise at first. You're going to want to use your legs and buttocks, instead of your abdominals. Stick with it; you'll get it!

Start by lying on your back, hands palm down at your sides, hips bent at right angles, knees slightly bent, ankles crossed. Keeping your shoulders and back down, exhale as you contract your abdominals to press your legs straight up, curling your pelvis like a scorpion curling its tail. It's a very small movement. Your legs and buttocks stay relaxed. Your legs shouldn't rock back and forth.

Start with one set of 5-8 reps. Work up to two sets of 10-15 reps.

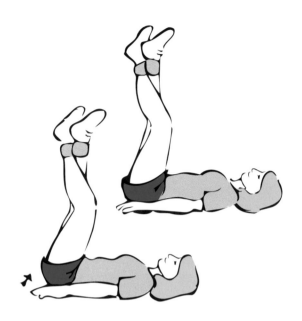

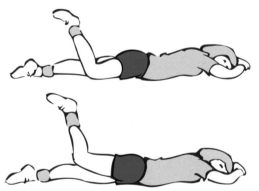

HIP EXTENSIONS
(Strengthens buttocks, backs of thighs)

Lie face down on the floor, resting your head on your hands as shown, legs fully extended. Keeping your upper body relaxed, exhale as you lift one leg straight up at the hip. It's a small movement of just a few inches. The knee is slightly flexed at the top of the movement. Inhale as you control the leg down. You should feel this in your buttocks and on the back of that thigh. Your shoulders and pelvis should stay pressed into the floor, don't rotate.

Start with one set of 5-8 reps with one leg, repeat to other side. Work up to two sets of 10-15 reps with each leg.

CONTRALATERAL ARM & LEG RAISE

(Whew, what a name! This one strengthens lower back, buttocks, shoulders, upper back)

Use the same starting position as for hip extensions, except that your arms are extended overhead. Again, this is a small movement, with no rotation.

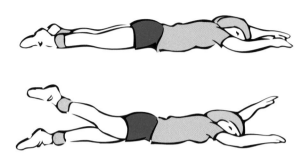

Exhale as you lift your left arm and right leg straight up. Shoulders and pelvis stay pressed into the floor. Don't try to lift either your arm or leg too far. Inhale as you control the movement down. Switch sides, using the right arm and left leg up.

Start with one set of 5-8 reps, alternating sides. Work up to two sets of 10-15 reps to each side.

If any of these exercises causes pain in a joint, like your knee, back or shoulder, stop that exercise and check with your doctor before you try it again.

Big Trouble

"Maggie, these exercises will make you stronger, and I bet they'll improve your posture and carriage. Once you can do two sets of 10-15 reps of each exercise, staying at that level will maintain your strength. And that's fine.

"Experts recommend that you give yourself at least a day of rest between doing strength exercises for any given muscle group. Since this entire strength routine will take you about 20-30 minutes, maximum, I encourage you to do all these exercises, two or three days a week. Remember to skip at least a day in between.

"If you decide that you want to get a bit stronger, then you need to increase the resistance, which means that you're going to need to start using weights, bands or other equipment. This is when I recommend that you consult with a qualified trainer, in your home or at a fitness center, to help you design that program."

"All right, I'll try these," Maggie said. "But if I end up looking like Arnold Schwarzenegger, you're in big trouble! Now, what about stretching? You said that's important, too."

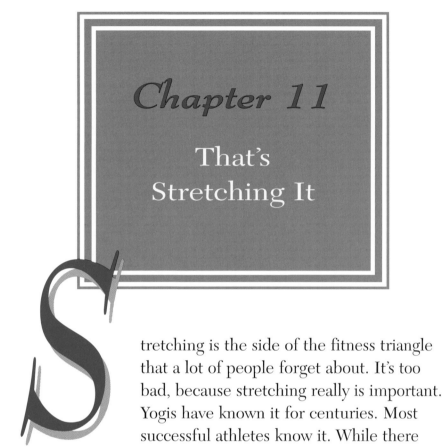

Chapter 11

That's Stretching It

Stretching is the side of the fitness triangle that a lot of people forget about. It's too bad, because stretching really is important. Yogis have known it for centuries. Most successful athletes know it. While there isn't a lot of research in this area, there is growing evidence that staying flexible has a number of benefits. Chief among these are:

- reduced risk of injury during recreational or performance activities

- improved performance during recreational or performance activities

- decreased muscle tension (stretching can be a great stress reducer—it just plain feels good!)

And that's just the beginning—many yoga experts believe that a variety of other benefits are experienced as well. The "mind-body" aspects of yoga may offer advantages ranging from improved focus and concentration to greater poise and calm to a variety of relaxing, stress-relieving qualities. Although these benefits have not been conclusively documented by western research, centuries of experience (plus growing popularity today) testify to the innate value of these stretches, which focus to a large extent on maintaining the flexibility of the spine.

A wide variety of yoga and yoga-based programs are available (ranging from the more traditional and eastern styles to the more contemporary western versions). Many people also enjoy the "gentle" nature of yoga (although some versions are extremely rigorous!) and find it a good way to reenter a fitness program, as well as a good way to balance their physical activities.

There are number of really great stretching programs available in fitness centers and on video. Most types of yoga, taught by a qualified instructor, offer great flexibility benefits. The Resources section lists some of the programs that I recommend.

What follows is a basic set of stretching exercises to get you started. They work. As with strength training, there are a lot of different opinions about the best way to stretch. I don't know that there is only one best way to stretch. I know that if I was working with you in person, I might do things a little differently than the guidelines I'm giving you in this book. My interest here is for you to have the lowest risk of overdoing it. I do know that if you follow these guidelines, you can become more flexible.

General Stretching Guidelines

- Move slowly to the "stretched" position, to the point where you feel a gentle tension, *not* pain, in the muscles being stretched.

- Hold the stretch for about 15 seconds, release, then repeat the stretch for another 15 seconds, release, then one or two more times. In other words, do 3-4 reps of each stretch, holding for about 15 seconds each time.

- Don't "bounce" in the stretched position. Hold a comfortable, steady position.

- Don't hold your breath. Maintain a comfortable breathing rhythm throughout all the stretches.

- Don't be surprised if you see different guidelines in other stuff you see or hear! That's okay.

BACKS OF THIGHS (HAMSTRINGS)
(Lying)

Lie on your back, one leg bent, foot flat on the floor. Keep the other leg straight, and lift it straight up, bending just at the hip. You can wrap your hands behind the thigh for support, but don't pull hard on that leg—just until you feel gentle tension in the hamstrings.

Repeat on the other side.

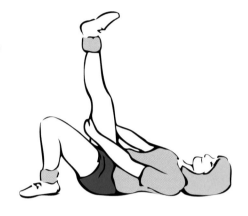

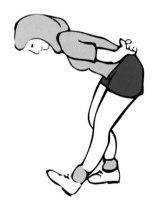

BACKS OF THIGHS (HAMSTRINGS)
(Standing)

This one's more difficult. Put one foot out in front of you, toes up. With your hands in the small of your back, bend the opposite knee and hip, not your lower back, until you feel the hamstrings stretch. The upper body comes forward, but it's at the hip. Head, neck and back stay in line.

146

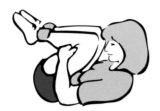

BUTTOCKS & LOWER BACK

Lie on your back and gently pull both legs to your chest clasping your hands between your thighs and calves. Curl your torso up toward your knees to increase the stretch.

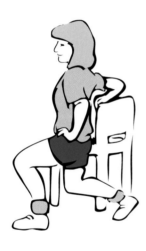

HIP FLEXORS

Use the same position as for the lunge in the last chapter. With one leg in front, the other behind, drop slowly straight toward the floor. Keep the front knee over that foot by bending the back knee. Feel the stretch in front of the hip closest to the chair. Repeat on the other side.

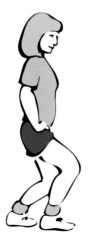

LOWER CALF AND ACHILLES

Start with hands on hips, one foot just slightly behind the other. Bend your knees and hips as you drop slowly straight toward the floor. Feel the stretch in the lower calf and Achilles tendon. Keep the upper body in good alignment and relaxed. Repeat on the other side.

UPPER CALF

Stand with hands on hips, one leg straight out behind you, heel down. Bend into the front knee, keeping head, neck, back and back leg in alignment, and keep the knee aligned over the foot. Don't arch your back. Feel the stretch in the upper calf area of the back leg. Repeat on the other side.

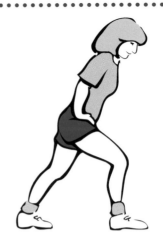

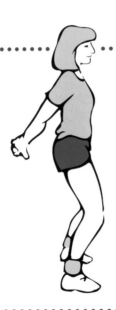

CHEST AND SHOULDERS

Standing with knees slightly flexed or sitting comfortably on a bench, reach behind your back at waist level, clasp your hands, palms facing your body, and press your arms up. Feel the stretch in the chest and fronts of shoulders.

FRONTS OF THIGHS (QUADRICEPS)

Holding the chair or a wall for support, bring one foot up behind you. Hold it with the same side hand, or a towel if your need to. Bend the opposite knee a little and gently pull your foot toward your buttocks, keeping the knee straight down to the floor.

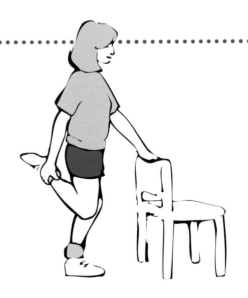

LOWER BACK

Lying on your back with both knees bent, hold your hands behind one thigh, and gently pull that leg toward your chest while you straighten the other leg. Repeat on the the other side.

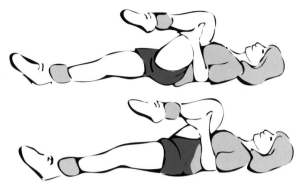

INNER THIGHS (ADDUCTORS)

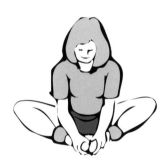

Sit comfortably on the floor (you might want to use a pillow at first), bend your knees and hips and bring the soles of your feet together in front of you as your knees drop open. Then bring your feet in toward you until you feel the stretch in the inner thighs. As you become more flexible, you can slowly round your torso forward.

These stretches will get you started. It should take you only about 10 minutes, at most, to do all of them. You can certainly do them 5 or 6 (or even 7) days a week if you want to. Just go slowly. These should leave you feeling relaxed and refreshed.

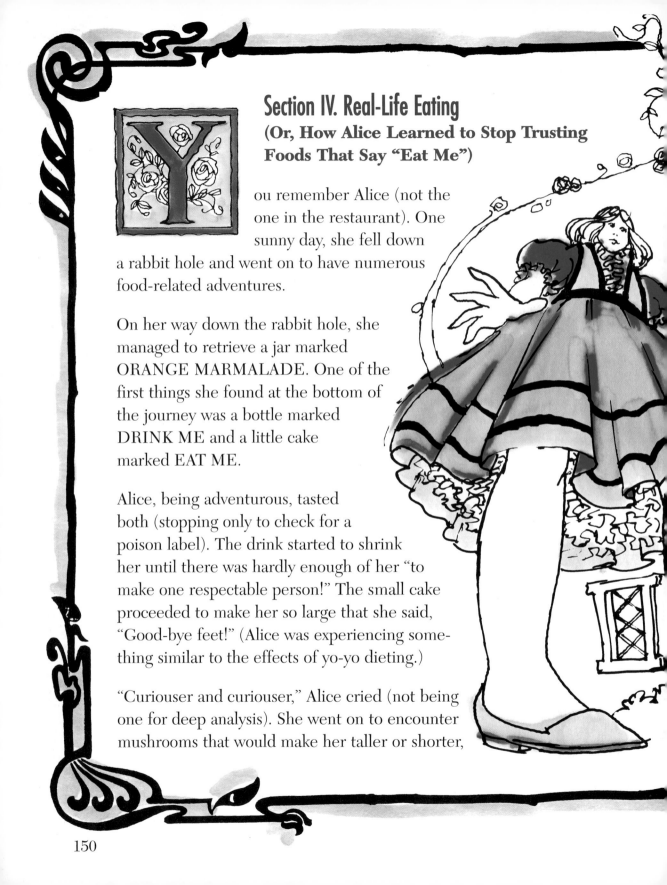

Section IV. Real-Life Eating
(Or, How Alice Learned to Stop Trusting Foods That Say "Eat Me")

You remember Alice (not the one in the restaurant). One sunny day, she fell down a rabbit hole and went on to have numerous food-related adventures.

On her way down the rabbit hole, she managed to retrieve a jar marked ORANGE MARMALADE. One of the first things she found at the bottom of the journey was a bottle marked DRINK ME and a little cake marked EAT ME.

Alice, being adventurous, tasted both (stopping only to check for a poison label). The drink started to shrink her until there was hardly enough of her "to make one respectable person!" The small cake proceeded to make her so large that she said, "Good-bye feet!" (Alice was experiencing something similar to the effects of yo-yo dieting.)

"Curiouser and curiouser," Alice cried (not being one for deep analysis). She went on to encounter mushrooms that would make her taller or shorter, a mad tea party, a duchess with a pepper problem, a queen obsessed with tarts, and a flying mock turtle preoccupied with lobster.

Not surprisingly (and like many of us who encounter the wonderland of food) Alice was left in quite a state of confusion, and ultimately wrote it all off as an odd dream. It is unclear whether the whole thing left her feeling hungry.

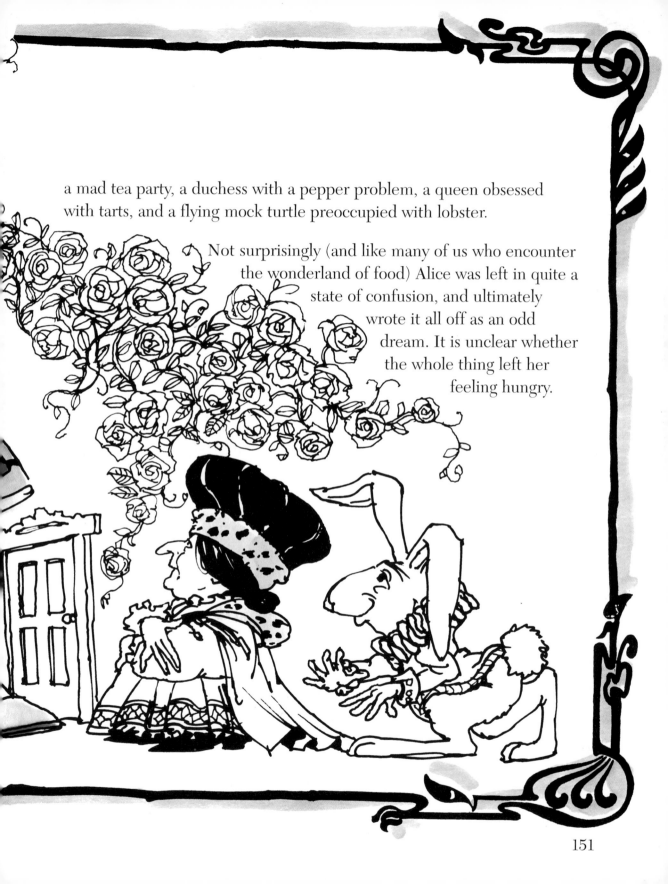

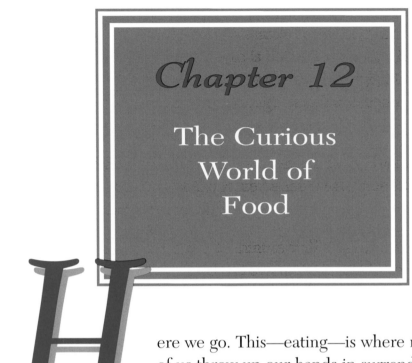

Chapter 12

The Curious World of Food

Here we go. This—eating—is where many of us throw up our hands in surrender. So many choices! So many foods begging "EAT ME!" And so much temptation to divide up things (it makes it seem simpler) as either "good" foods (healthy, dull, unsatisfying) or "bad" foods (sinful, delicious, thrilling). We also tend to believe that we are all created equal—that choosing certain foods is equally simple or difficult for all of us, and our bodies respond in pretty much the same ways to all foods (some foods will make us big, and others will make us shrink). But in the wonderland of food, things are not always as they seem. Or, as Jack Nicholson expressed so vividly in *The Shining*, "All work ('good' foods) and no play ('bad' foods) makes Jack a dull boy." (I threw in the food part, but if you've ever been going crazy on a restrictive diet, you may be able to relate to that character!)

For one thing, foods can pretend on their labels—through the miracle of advertising—to be better than they really are. A lot of foods pretend to be worse than they really are (appealing to our rebel side) when it is only consistently large quantities that could be trouble.

For another thing, food preferences are a tricky thing. New (early) research tells us there are chemicals in the body that may regulate at least some of our individual preferences for carbohydrates and fats—some of us may be "wired" for wanting more of one or the other (challenging the allegation that our food preferences are based solely on greed, lack of willpower, etc.). This process that regulates our appetites is not a simple one, any more than are the metabolic processes that regulate how our bodies use food and nutrients.

Finally, how each of us responds to various dietary habits is unique. I'll illustrate with another story:

Once upon a time there was a little lady, Mrs. Boote, who lived in a shoe—a very big shoe. Her husband traveled a lot, selling various and sundry gadgets throughout the kingdom, but over the years they had eight children, four girls and four boys. And during the years when all eight kids were hanging around the shoe, mealtime was almost a constant process.

Mrs. Boote was concerned that she might not be feeding her family as well as she should: There was so much confusing information about good nutrition. The village baker said you should eat lots of this. The village butcher said you should eat lots of that. And the village cobbler said, "No, they're both wrong. You don't really need very much of this and that. What you really need is a lot of the-other-thing."

This, that or the-other-thing—who was she supposed to

believe? To top it all off, the king's wizard had just sent out a flyer saying that he'd come up with a new magic potion everyone should get. He was certain that this potion would provide the kingdom's residents with sure protection against a number of troublesome maladies. *"Hmm, that's what he said the last time he came up with a new potion,"* thought Mrs. Boote to herself.

Besides it was expensive, at least for Mrs. Boote, trying to manage a food budget for ten people. It seemed like her family was relatively healthy, and her kids were all growing fine. So, Mrs. Boote decided that she'd just have to keep feeding her family pretty much as she had been: lots of vegetables and fruits (when in season), bread with flour that the baker ground on his stone mill, porridge with beans and potatoes and a little bit of lamb from the butcher. With her limited budget, she couldn't afford a lot of meat. And they got cheese when they could—but it was kind of a treat.

As the kids grew up, and one by one left the shoe to make their own way in the world, Mrs. Boote felt good, knowing that the way she fed her family couldn't have been too bad. Nothing too fancy or complicated, mostly just common sense.

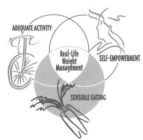

But one thing was always curious to Mrs. Boote. *"Why,"* she wondered to herself, *"are three of them somewhat portly, three pretty average size, and two thin, even though I feed all the kids the same way and they're all pretty active?"*

I guess genetics was at work even during Mrs. Boote's time!

No, It Isn't Easy!

A lot of emphasis has been put on low-fat eating, to the point where some people believe that fat content matters but overall quantity of food doesn't. Others believe that it is strictly calorie-counting that makes the difference, regardless of the kinds of food. You can probably guess what I'm going to tell you: Both attitudes are extreme and neither is accurate! Quantity of food and quality of food both "matter." There is no easy answer, as much as we might wish for one!

You are going to find that this section on healthy eating is relatively short, straightforward, and primarily educational. This is a deliberate choice, for several reasons:

- Too much damage has already been done by making nutrition much more complicated and confusing than it needs to be.

- Because the focus has been on weight loss, pitching programs and misinformation, the basic educational element of nutrition has been lacking. Consequently, there are some nutrition fundamentals that are not commonly understood by most people. Yet these are the principles which can easily guide your food choices in a more healthy direction.

- The key challenge for healthy eating, as with physical activity, is not learning what you need to do, but motivating yourself to do it—and do it permanently. (We will talk more about this at the end of this section.)

I am not going to pretend that mastering the art of food choices is an easy one, nor will I encourage you to believe that dramatic changes are well within your reach at this moment. (As I said before, even your ability to make behavior changes is somewhat impacted by genetics.) What I *will* say is that trying—even slowly—to find some middle ground between a restrictive, unhealthy war with food and an I-give-up-anything-goes guilty dance with food is well worth the effort.

Finding a way to make more sensible food choices instead of extreme ones, combined with an active lifestyle and a self-empowering approach to the process, is going to greatly change your health risk profile, not to mention the quality of your life—and last but not least, your body.

The "Sensible" Word

"You've used the phrase *sensible eating* so many times," Maggie said to me at our next appointment, "I'd like to know what you mean by it. I'm confused about what makes up a good diet. One expert says I should eat lots of carbohydrates, just a little protein and hardly any fat all. The next book I pick up is by another expert who tells me that to lose weight I should eat his 14-day plan which has me practically eliminate carbohydrates, but be sure to take supplements.

"Another one says I shouldn't eat proteins and carbohydrates at the same meal because my digestive system can't handle it. But I found out that almost all foods have some protein and carbohydrate, so all I could eat is meat or oils. Then someone else comes along with a nutritional program supposedly based on the latest research. He tells me that the food I buy at the grocery store is so depleted of nutrients that I need to spend about $100 a month, just for me, if I want to be adequately nourished. The price goes up to several hundred dollars a month just for pills and powders if I get the program for Jim and the kids, as well. This salesman follows the program, and boy has his energy level gone up. Besides that, he said I can also sell the product and make a lot of money; then it won't cost me anything!"

"Just out of curiosity, how are you making your food choices right now?" I asked. I was pretty sure I knew what her response would be—and I was right.

"Frankly, I've given up on the whole thing," she told me. "I'm not really making choices—I'm just going with what I feel like."

"Maggie, I can understand your frustration. I hear it from a lot of people—they're tired of all the plans and programs. The choices were so confusing that they stopped making choices and went back to what I call letting the food choose them—based on what looks good or smells good at the moment. Research shows that taste is the number one reason for food choices. Before we go any further, let me give you some information about the basic principles of nutrition."

The Basics

Basic nutrition doesn't have to be confusing. As I mentioned, however, there are some key fundamentals to basic nutrition that most of us don't understand very well—and they could make our food choices and weight management efforts a whole lot easier. You may find that you are familiar with some of the concepts that follow, but read carefully: You are likely to find some surprising (and useful) new facts.

All the foods we eat are made up of various combinations of the six basic nutrients: carbohydrates, fats, proteins, vitamins, minerals and water. In fact, that's what our body is made of as well! Most foods have some of all the nutrients, just in different percentages. Let's briefly go through all six.

Carbohydrates

Carbohydrates (carbs) are a primary source of energy for the cells in your body—brain cells, muscle cells, and so on. The carbohydrate family includes both complex carbohydrates (starch), and simple sugars, like fructose and glucose. Complex carbs are nothing more than a whole bunch of simple sugars all bound together. The body converts all the carbs we eat into glucose, which the cells then use to make energy.

Interestingly, we don't store very much glucose in our body —some in the liver and some in the muscles, but not a whole lot more. It's important to eat adequate carbs every day to replace what's used up making energy. The more active you are, the more carbs you need.

Grains, vegetables, legumes (beans and peas), fruits and even milk are good sources of complex carbohydrates.

"My body uses sugar to make energy?" Maggie asks. "So why don't I just eat a lot of candy and soda, instead of this stuff about eating mostly complex carbs?"

"Good question. I'm not going to go too deeply into the chemistry involved. Essentially, if you eat a lot of simple sugar all at once, your blood sugar level rises rapidly. Then your pancreas secretes a bunch of the hormone insulin, to bring the blood sugar level back down. Two potential problems:

- Since you can use only a certain amount of glucose at a time, if the blood sugar level is too high, insulin starts a process whereby some of the glucose is changed to fat and stored in a fat cell.

- The rapid rise in blood sugar likely causes too much insulin to be released, resulting a couple of hours later in a temporarily low blood sugar level. The brain senses this, leading to a potential craving for more sugar.

Complex carbs are kind of like a time-release pill. When you eat complex carbs, you don't have a whole bunch of simple sugar enter the bloodstream all at once. Instead, complex carbs are digested in the intestines, with the simple sugar building blocks entering the bloodstream over a much longer period of time. Plus, if you eat a variety of foods high in complex carbs, you're getting a lot of other nutrients. The *only* nutrient in the soda is sugar.

Most experts recommend that we get between 60-65% of our daily calories from carbs, mostly the complex kind.

Fats

Fats, like carbs, come in two major varieties, saturated and unsaturated. And, also like carbs, the primary purpose of fat is energy production.

Animal foods, in general, provide fats which are mostly saturated. Red meats, poultry (especially the skin), lamb, pork, and dairy have mostly saturated fat. Surprisingly, so do tropical oils, like coconut and palm oil. Fish, and vegetable oils provide mostly unsaturated fats. Research tells us that we should cut back on saturated fats since they're the ones which increase the risk of heart disease and certain cancers.

That's why skim or 1% milk, and low-fat cheeses and yogurt are a healthier choice than whole milk products. Cooking with oils—olive, sesame, safflower, canola—is a healthier method than cooking with butter or shortening made from animal fat.

When a highly unsaturated oil, like corn oil, is made into margarine, it changes to being much more like a saturated fat. The harder the margarine, the more highly saturated its fat content. Soft, tub margarine is a healthier choice than the harder, stick variety.

Keep one thing in mind—most of the fat you consume should be unsaturated, but both types of fat have exactly the same number of calories. And fat has more than twice as many calories per ounce as carbohydrate. We don't need to eat very much fat, of any kind! About 20-25% of daily calories is the typical recommendation. The American Heart Association says no more than 30%. Fat is not "bad." We need some. It's just that it's pretty easy to get too much.

Proteins

Proteins are used mainly for providing the structure for the many cells and tissues in the body. They also are used in the immune system, to transport vital elements in the bloodstream, and to make up many of the hormones, like insulin. There are thousands of different kinds of proteins, all made from building blocks called amino acids, eight of which we must get in our diet (the essential amino acids).

Animal foods provide us with all of the essential amino acids. They are called complete proteins. Plant foods, which lack one or more of the essential amino acids, are incomplete proteins. Including some animal food in your diet is an easy way to ensure that you're getting complete proteins, as well as other vital nutrients like vitamin B12.

However, combining grains and legumes—rice and beans, for example—also provides complete proteins. (I've listed a couple of books in the Resources section which go into detail regarding vegetarian eating.)

Since protein is such a vital part of our body, some people think we need to eat a lot of protein. That doesn't seem to be the case. About 10-15% of daily calories is the general recommendation. Another reference is about one-half gram of protein daily for each pound of body weight.

Vitamins and Minerals

Vitamins and minerals are essential for the proper working of the body's multitude of functions. For example, the B vitamins are necessary to help use glucose for making energy. Calcium is not only essential for strong bones and teeth, but it also plays an integral role in muscle contraction. Whole books are written just on the role of these two nutrients, so check out the sources in the Resource section if you want more information.

"I just want to know if I need vitamin and mineral supplements?" That's Maggie's question, and a lot of other people's, as well.

To be honest, I don't really know. In a survey of registered dietitians, reported in the *Nutrition Desk Reference*, half said they recommend supplements, half said that if you eat a good diet you don't need them. All the information on the anti-oxidant vitamins (beta-carotene, and vitamins C and E) has led many researchers and practitioners to recommend that we take supplements of them. But other experts, equally knowledgeable and qualified, say no, it's too early to tell. Just eat a good diet.

Here's my recommendation. (It's what I do.) Try to use the 80/20 approach with the specific guidelines in the next chapter. In general, for now, focus your attention on eating a wide variety of different foods, with the majority coming from whole grains, vegetables, fruits and legumes. Include some low-fat dairy, fish, a little meat if you want, some oils and a few treats. Most important, eat enough to give your body the nutrients it needs.

And most days (when I remember!), I take a broad-spectrum multivitamin/mineral supplement you can get at most any drug store or supermarket. I look at it as sort of an insurance policy, in case I might not be getting enough in my diet. I check the label to see that none of the nutrients comes in excess of about 150% of the recommended daily requirement. I'm not aware of any unbiased evidence that the extra expensive supplements are any better than the "store bought" kind.

I'm going to keep my eyes and ears open on the anti-oxidant research. For now I'm trying to make sure I get plenty of:

- citrus fruits and juices for vitamin C

- orange and dark green vegetables for beta-carotene

and

- sweet potatoes and sunflower seeds for vitamin E.

Women need to be especially attentive to getting adequate calcium, iron and, if you're thinking about getting pregnant or are pregnant or nursing, folic acid (also called folate). You're at the greatest risk of not getting enough if you're eating a low calorie diet, which is less than 1,200 calories a day.

To meet women's nutritional needs, I recommend:

- Eat at least 1,200 calories a day!

- Include 3 glasses of skim milk, or 3 servings of non-fat yogurt (for calcium).

- Drink some orange juice with the meal which has some animal food (vitamin C helps iron absorption, and has a good amount of folic acid).

- Eat more lentils and spinach (both excellent sources of folic acid).

- You might also consider taking a supplement which includes a little more of these nutrients.

I encourage you to talk with your physician or a registered dietitian with any questions about your specific needs.

Can you eat a lousy diet and make up for it by taking supplements?

No.

Do I give my kids a vitamin/mineral supplement?

Yes, because I know they don't always eat enough fruits and vegetables!

Water

Water is a nutrient? Yes, and an incredibly important one. Twenty-four hours a day—waking, sleeping, exercising— your body is losing water in its attempt to regulate your internal temperature. The heat that's produced as a by-product of energy production in your body (just like heat is a by-product when your car's engine burns gasoline to make energy) is released outside your body through sweat and water vapor in your breath.

You might not think you're sweating while you watch TV. You are. It's just that the sweat evaporates before it gets to your skin. When you start exercising, muscles make a lot more energy, a lot more heat is produced, and the water loss increases considerably.

You can see the water vapor in your breath on a cold day. When you start exercising, you obviously breathe faster and more deeply, further adding to water loss.

You need to drink a lot of water even if you just sit around all day. You need to really increase your water intake when you start becoming more active.

Drink at least eight glasses of water a day, in addition to the fruit and veggie juices you may consume in moderation. But space it out. Like most things, a little bit at a time is better than all at once. If you down three glasses full in short order, it puts a whole lot of water into the bloodstream at once. This sends the kidneys into overdrive, and you to the bathroom.

If you spread those three glasses out over a couple of hours, it allows more of the water to go from the bloodstream into the cells, where it's needed—and not so much into your bladder, where it's not.

With regard to water needs and exercise, the research suggests that we:

- Drink about 8-10 ounces (about one glass) of water in the half-hour before the exercise session.

- Drink 3-4 ounces every 10 minutes during exercise, and then another 8-10 ounces in the half-hour following the session. The harder you work, the more water you need.

- Don't depend on your sense of thirst to tell you when you need water. By the time we humans are thirsty, we're already somewhat dehydrated. Develop the habit of drinking more water.

"How about all these sports drinks?" Maggie wonders. "Do I need them?"

"Unless your exercise session is going to last for more than an hour to an hour and half, no. What you need is water. If your session lasts longer, then, yes, you do need something to give you some glucose. Those drinks are one way to do that."

"How about those rubber belts I've seen advertised to shrink my waist and thighs three inches during an exercise session? Do they really work?"

"Yes, you'll lose some inches during a workout, because those belts increase the water loss in those areas. Is it fat loss? No. Will you regain those inches as soon as you replace the water that was lost? Yes. And don't ever exercise in a rubberized sweat suit. Sweat releases heat only when it evaporates. Those suits prevent the evaporation, and can lead to a dangerous elevation in your body temperature."

There you have it. Basic nutrition. That wasn't so bad, was it? Carbohydrates, fats, proteins, vitamins, minerals and water. Now let's see how they all fit together in this "sensible diet" I've been recommending.

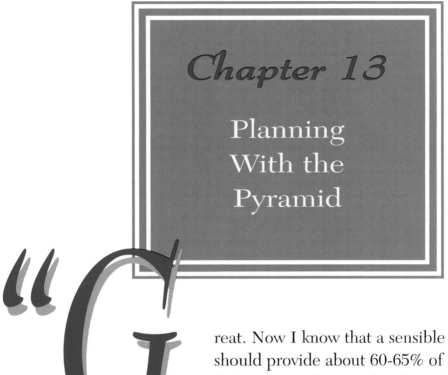

Chapter 13

Planning With the Pyramid

"Great. Now I know that a sensible diet should provide about 60-65% of my daily calories from carbs, about 20-25% from fat and about 10-15% from protein," said Maggie, with a little sarcasm. "But that really doesn't mean very much to me. I don't know the percentage of carbs, fats and proteins in the foods that I eat. Sure, I know some foods are high in fat, some are high in carbs, and some are good sources of protein. But I'm not interested in having to look at charts and tables which give me the grams of this and grams of that, and then calculating all that stuff. Isn't there an easier way to know that I'm eating a healthy diet?"

"I think so. It won't be absolutely precise, but it'll work. Some people do want to keep precise records and calculate, or have a computer calculate, a comprehensive dietary record. But Maggie, I think a lot of people share your feelings. They would like to eat a healthy diet, but they don't want to weigh and measure everything they eat, either. But I will ask you to keep some records, like a journal. It's great feedback. It'll take a little time and effort, especially at first. But it's not very detailed and it won't take you very long."

80/20 and the Pyramid

The U.S. Department of Agriculture recently spearheaded a major project to make it easier for the public to know what they should be eating. The result is the Food Guide Pyramid. For most people, it's a lot more practical and easy to understand than trying to calculate the percentages of carbs, fat and protein.

If you eat according to the guidelines given in the pyramid, it's very likely that you'll be well within the recommended percentages. That's the way it has been designed. You can also determine your caloric intake in a general and easy way based on the recommendations of the pyramid. (We'll talk about that later.) This is one useful pyramid!

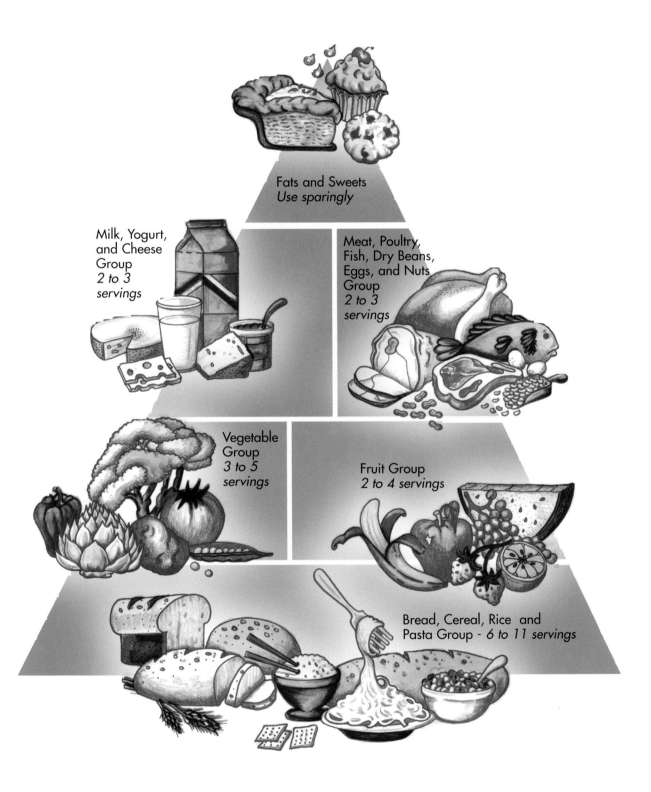

Fats and Sweets
Use sparingly

Milk, Yogurt, and Cheese Group
2 to 3 servings

Meat, Poultry, Fish, Dry Beans, Eggs, and Nuts Group
2 to 3 servings

Vegetable Group
3 to 5 servings

Fruit Group
2 to 4 servings

Bread, Cereal, Rice and Pasta Group - *6 to 11 servings*

Now I'll finally answer Maggie's question, "What is a sensible diet?" It's a long sentence, but here it goes: A sensible daily diet is one which, *at least 80% of the time*, provides 6-11 servings from the bread, cereal, rice and pasta group; 3-5 servings from the vegetable group; 2-4 servings from the fruit group; 2-3 servings from the milk, yogurt and cheese group; 2-3 servings from the meat, poultry, fish, dry beans, eggs and nuts group; and not very much from the fats and sweets group.

If you *don't* match these daily servings 20% of the time or less, I personally don't think it's that big of a deal.

Clearly, I'm not recommending that you go out one day a week and totally gorge yourself—waiting with anxious anticipation the whole week for that day when you can go off your diet! That wouldn't be very healthy. And you probably wouldn't stick with this approach any longer than some of the other approaches you've tried.

The 80/20 approach to using the pyramid is a lifestyle. Hopefully you can use it for the rest of your life. It means that if you want to go to a Sunday morning buffet brunch, do it. And don't feel guilty about it.

Or if you go to a friend's house for dinner and you're served barbecue ribs, enjoy them. And don't feel guilty about it.

It simply means that you're not going to approach your eating plan from the extremes: always/never, good/bad. Unless you're allergic to it, I can't think of any one food you should never eat. Nor can I think of any one food that you should always eat.

Rather than classifying foods as good or bad, how about classifying them as high in complex carbs, low in fat, high in fat, high in sugar, good sources of protein?

Almost anything you eat has some nutritional value. If it's high in fat or sugar, don't eat very much of it. That's at the top of the pyramid and there's not much room up there! There *is* lots of room, however, for foods high in complex carbs. Good protein foods have quite a bit of space as well.

Maggie asked me why fats get so much less room that foods high in protein, even though the recommended intake as a percent of total calories is nearly the same. It's because fat has more than twice as many calories per ounce as protein or carbs. You don't have to eat very much fat to get a lot of calories.

How Much is a Serving?

Let's look at each section of the pyramid to see how much food you actually need to eat to match the serving recommendation.

Bread, Cereal, Rice and Pasta Group

6-11 servings. (This group also includes grains such as barley and millet.)

An easy way to remember how much one serving is:

- 1 ounce (about a cup) packaged breakfast cereal

- 1/2 cup cooked rice, cereal or pasta

- 1 slice of bread

6-11 servings might sound like a lot, but let's see…

> *Breakfast*
>
> | | |
> |---|---|
> | Bowl of packaged cereal (2 cups) | 2 servings |
>
> *Lunch*
>
> | | |
> |---|---|
> | Sandwich, 2 slices of bread | 2 servings |
>
> *Dinner*
>
> | | |
> |---|---|
> | Pasta (1-1/2 cups) | 3 servings |
>
> *Snack*
>
> | | |
> |---|---|
> | Pretzels | 1 serving |
> | *TOTAL =* | 8 servings |

It's not that difficult to get the 6-11 servings. But there are a few really important things to keep in mind:

- This group also includes the pastries, cookies, cakes, etc., which are made from white flour. These will definitely count as servings, but they are also usually made with fat and sugar. Lots of calories per serving!

- You'll get a lot more fiber if you eat whole grains rather than refined flour. Whole grain breads and cereals are excellent nutrition sources.

- The pasta is usually pretty low in fat, but the sauce may not be. Try to use tomato based sauces as much as possible. If you use meat in the sauce, use lean cuts.

- Lots of packaged cereals are loaded with sugar. When you read the label, ideally most of the carbohydrates should come from starch, not sugar.

Vegetable Group

3-5 servings

One serving is...

- 1 cup raw leafy vegetables

- 1/2 cup other veggies, cooked or raw

- 3/4 cup vegetable juice.

How hard is it to get 3-5 servings?

Lunch

1 carrot	1 serving
Lettuce, onion, tomato	1 serving
(on a sandwich)	

Dinner

1/2 cup broccoli	1 serving
1/2 cup corn	1 serving

Snack

6 ounces tomato juice	1 serving
TOTAL =	5 servings

As with the bread group, keep in mind that it's what you put on the vegetables that can really add up the calories. Try using light margarine instead of butter, lemon juice or spices instead of rich cream or cheese sauces. If you use the sauce, just use a little bit for taste. Don't smother the veggies!

Fruit Group

2-4 servings

One serving is...

- 1 medium sized apple, orange, banana, peach or pear

- 1 cup chopped, cooked or canned fruit

- 1 cup raspberries, strawberries

- 6 ounces fruit juice

Is it easy to get your servings? Yes.

Breakfast

Banana on cereal	1 serving
6 ounces orange juice	1 serving

Afternoon snack

Apple	1 serving

Evening snack

1 cup grapes	1 serving
TOTAL =	4 servings

Fruit is excellent as a pick-me-up snack. And drinking fruit juice is an easy way to get your daily servings. But be careful—one medium orange has about 60 calories, where-as 8 ounces of orange juice has about 110 calories. Don't drink juice instead of water. Juice is a food.

When buying canned fruit, look for the ones that are canned "in their own juice" not the ones which are canned "in heavy syrup." Syrup is just more sugar.

Meat, Poultry, Fish, Dry Beans, Eggs and Nuts Group

2-3 servings

One serving is…

- 3 eggs (if you eat an egg, that's 1/3 of a serving)

- 1 cup cooked beans

- 3 ounces cooked fish

- 3 ounces beef, chicken or pork

- 1 cup dry roasted nuts (but there's over 800 calories!)

I think it's pretty obvious how easy it is to get your recommended servings from this group! Many Americans get way more than the recommendation.

Additionally, many of these foods are high in saturated fat.

Here are some tips:

- Take the skin off chicken and turkey before you eat the meat.

175

- Choose lean cuts of beef and pork, like flank, round or loin.

- Trim all visible fat.

- Broil or bake, rather than frying.

- A typical restaurant steak is 6-8 ounces. As a reference for how big a 3-ounce serving is, a deck of cards is about the size of three ounces of meat (especially useful if you're a gambler!).

Milk, Yogurt and Cheese Group

2-3 servings

One serving is…

- 8 ounces milk

- 8 ounces yogurt

- 2 cups cottage cheese

- 1 cup ice cream

- 2 ounces processed cheese

- 1 ounce natural cheese

Dairy Intake Recommendations:

- Use skim milk or 1% milk and milk products. You get all the nutrients found in whole milk, without the saturated fat.

- Same with yogurt. Use the lowfat yogurt. But many also have a lot of added sugar. Read the label.

- 12 ounces of premium ice cream has about 525 calories! How easily can you pay for it in your energy bank?

Fats, Oils and Sweets

There are no recommendations for the number of daily servings you should get from this group. You know it shouldn't be very much, at least most of the time.

Common Sense

"You know," Maggie tells me when we finish going through each group in the pyramid, "I really knew most of this stuff already. Sometimes it's hard to know exactly how many servings to put into each group, like if I have a chicken Caesar salad. But I can probably make a pretty good guess based on the size of the salad. Obviously, with the dressing, I've made a contribution to the fats and oils group."

"A lot of it's just common sense, isn't it?"

"I'd have to say yes. I think it is. If we know that most of our daily foods should come from grains, veggies, and fruits, less from meats and dairy, and not much at all from fats and sweets, it's not that hard to see if our diet matches that general scheme."

Variety is important to most people. Eating the same things day after day is not appealing to most of us. In many parts of the world, there isn't a lot of choice. But the food choices in most technologically developed countries are unbelievable in comparison. Unfortunately, many of the choices are high fat, high sugar, low nutritional value.

If you're interested, there are number of excellent books and products available which give you a multitude of different recipes that will keep you right in line with the pyramid's guidelines. I've listed some of my favorites in the Resources section.

What I'd like to do now is take the information on the number of servings and serving sizes, and translate it to match various calorie levels.

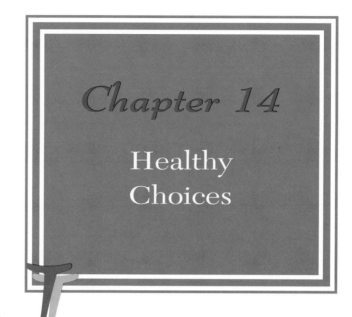

Chapter 14

Healthy Choices

Now that you've got some idea of the relative number of servings from each group of foods you should eat, let's see what that means in relation to actual meals. Keep in mind that within each major food group, there can be a lot of difference in the number of calories you'll get from a single serving of one food compared with a single serving of another food.

For example, within the meat group a single serving of three ounces of roasted chicken breast (without the skin) provides 147 calories. A single serving of three ounces of lean, broiled beef sirloin provides 229 calories.

In the dairy food group, a serving of 8 ounces of skim milk has 86 calories, 8 ounces of whole milk (4% milkfat) has 150 calories.

One carrot—that's one serving of vegetables—has about 35 calories. Ten french fries (also one serving) has 160 calories. When was the last time you saw anyone eat just 10 french fries?

Sounds like the potato chip commercial: Try to eat just one. You can probably guess what the calorie story is with potato chips! I read somewhere that what they should be called is fat chips, with a little potato added.

One apple, a serving of fruit, 80 calories. Ten dried dates, also a serving, 230 calories.

Same story with the bread group. A plain English muffin, one serving, 60 calories. One small danish pastry, one serving, 125 calories.

In other words, all single servings are not created equal with regard to calorie content.

A Word on Calories

My experience tells me that trying to match yourself with a specific daily calorie plan doesn't work for most of us, at least not for long. I used to recommend daily eating plans built around a set number of calories. I don't anymore. They seldom worked.

Daily calorie plans can encourage you to focus too much of your attention on how many calories you're eating, and tempt you to lose focus of the fact that getting as active as you can is the real key. It's back to that old control thing. Real-life weight management is about not having to feel the need for so much control because you're making healthy choices in your life—both in activity and in food.

Some long-distance endurance athletes—cyclists, cross-country skiers, runners—need to eat 4,000 or more calories a day in order to give their bodies the nutrients necessary to make the energy required for their events. Of course, when they stop competing, they need to reduce their calories or they'll quickly build up a big energy reserve in their fat cells!

If you need to lose some weight, your first thought should be, *"How can I add some more activity to my lifestyle?"* Then, consider your diet as an adjunct. I recommend a general plan of trying to match your eating with the pyramid's guidelines. I'll show you how to develop that sensible eating plan in the next chapter.

For those of you who are concerned about the portions you are eating, and would like to know specific calorie information, that's fine, too. As long as you promise me that you won't become so focused on it that you can't wait until you're done with this latest calorie-counting diet! The Resources section includes some books and software that you can use to figure out your daily calories.

Get Real is *not* a low calorie diet plan. It's a lifestyle plan to help you become healthier. Its focus is on accepting yourself for who you are, *getting more active*, and eating sensibly. The sample daily servings at various calorie levels are included to help you gain some understanding and develop some new lifetime eating habits.

One important suggestion: If you're going to reduce your daily calorie intake, don't do it in any greater than 500 calorie per day increments. There's pretty strong evidence that if you make greater than 500 calorie per day decreases too rapidly, the "set point" may slow your metabolism as a protection against what it senses as inadequate calories.

Spacing out the decrease appears to reduce the chances of that happening.

Servings in the Pyramid

Here are some examples of how you could meet the pyramid's recommendations at a number of different daily calorie intakes. I include this in order for you to get a general idea of serving sizes and food choices that go along with various calorie intakes. It is not necessary or even desirable for you to count every calorie you eat—it is, however, useful to have a general idea of where your calorie intake is today, in case you want to adjust that amount in a given direction at some point.

As I mentioned before, although continuous calorie counting is not often a practical or effective method, *quantity* of food *is* a weight management factor—although it is certainly not the only one.

Number of Daily Servings from Each Pyramid Group

Daily Intake	1600 Calories	2200 Calories	2800 Calories
Breads group	6	9	11
Vegetables group	3	4	5
Fruits group	2	3	4
Meats group	2	2	2-3
Dairy group	2-3	2-3	2-3

Additional daily and weekly eating plan examples from Maggie's experience, followed by forms you can use, are included in the final section of this book.

Long-term Success

Research suggests that regular exercise, not dieting or even dieting with exercise, is the key to keeping the weight off. Dr. Foreyt reports that in a two-year study of three groups—one who dieted only, one who combined diet with exercise, and one who exercised only—the group that focused on exercise was the only group to successfully maintain weight loss after two years. Fascinating!

It's not surprising that the group which only restricted calories wasn't successful in the long run. But the diet and exercise group's results are very interesting. It seems that because they considered the diet and exercise regimens to be like a partnership, when they couldn't handle the forced diet any longer, they also gave up the exercise.

Here's the take-home lesson: Don't force yourself into a diet and exercise program. And don't consider a diet and exercise program as dependent on one another with a distinct "end point." If it's not something you think you can live with for the rest of your life, obviously you're not going to live with it for the rest of your life!

Focus on getting more active and cutting back on the fat in your diet. If you're like most people, forcing yourself into a highly controlled calorie plan won't work for very long. And if you tie a restricted calorie diet to an exercise program, when you quit the diet, you'll probably also quit the exercise program.

Here are some additional ways to cut back on dietary fat and reduce the risk of overeating.

Label Reading

Food manufacturers are now required to put a nutrition label on almost all food products. Reading the labels can help you immensely in your quest to reduce the number of fat calories in your daily diet. Here's an example:

"Maggie," I asked, "you have a choice between two different types of snacks, 5/8 of an ounce of potato chips (a very small bag!) or four ounces of nonfat fruit yogurt. How can you use the labels to help you pick the snack lowest in fat and highest in other nutrients?"

Maggie looked at the labels:

<u>Potato Chips</u>

Serving Size: 5/8 ounce

Total Calories: 90

Total Fat: 5 grams

Fat Calories: 45 (5 grams x 9 calories/gram of fat)

Total Carbohydrate: 10 grams

Total Protein: 1 gram

<u>Nonfat Fruit Yogurt</u>

Serving Size: 4 ounces

Total Calories: 100

Total Fat: 0 grams

Fat Calories: 0

Total Carbohydrate: 21 grams (19 from sugar)

Total Protein: 5 grams

"Well, let's see," Maggie said. "I see from the label that the yogurt has calcium and vitamin C, so it's obviously a more nutritious snack. The chips are about 50% fat calories. The yogurt is 0% fat calories. Plus, I get almost eight times more food (4 ounces v. 5/8 ounce.) So...I can probably eat as much of the yogurt as I want, right?"

I told Maggie she was right to read the labels and that yogurt is definitely the more nutritious snack. "But," I added, "keep two things in mind. The fact that the yogurt doesn't have fat doesn't mean that you can eat unlimited quantities. It still has 100 calories per serving. This is one of the misconceptions about low-fat foods. Sure, they're often healthful, but *they still contain calories*. Some people have assumed that as long as they eat low-fat foods, they can consume unlimited amounts. Not true!

"This is probably a big part of the reason why those who have significantly cut back on dietary fat but consumed large quantities of low-fat foods have not realized any weight loss—or perhaps have even gained weight. The energy balance relationship still holds, regardless of where the calories come from.

"Second, if you want to have a few potato chips once in a while, do it. Just realize that you're getting a lot of calories and very little nutrient value."

Here's another question: Are all high-fat foods to be avoided?

My answer is No. For example:

<u>Peanuts</u>

Serving Size: 1/2 ounce (very small bag)

Total Calories: 90

Total Fat: 7 grams

Fat Calories: 63

Total Carbohydrate: 4 grams

Total Protein: 3 grams

Are peanuts high in fat? Yes. Are peanuts "bad food"? No. They are a source of protein, as well as some other nutrients. Should you eat very many of them? No. Not unless you're a competitive endurance athlete who needs to eat 4,000 or more calories a day!

You Make the Choice

Here's another example of comparing about the same amount of food, but considering the tremendous difference in the number of calories.

For lunch:

option 1	approx. calories
Cheeseburger (on a bun, lettuce, onions, pickles, tomato, mayo)	450
Large fries	400
Regular milkshake	<u>400</u>
TOTAL =	1,250

option 2	
Turkey breast sandwich (whole wheat bread, lettuce, onions, pickles, tomato, 1 tsp. non-fat mayo)	400
8 oz. glass of 1% milk, blended with strawberries	110
2 ounces pretzels (small bag)	<u>100</u>
TOTAL =	610

Pretty dramatic difference. For about the same amount of food, you get twice as many calories with option 1. Is one choice wrong and one right? No. Is one choice lower in calories and much lower in fat? Yes. You're the one who needs to decide which one you want to choose.

Eating Throughout the Day

It is becoming more and more evident that eating throughout the day is an important aspect of a sensible nutrition lifestyle. The reasons are pretty clear:

1. If you get about 75% of your calories before your evening meal (or the meal before you go to sleep if you work at night), you have a much lower chance of binging on large volumes of food. What seems to be going on is that if you deprive yourself of calories throughout the day, your endocrine system (the one that deals with hormones) ends up sending powerful messages from the brain's eating centers to your appetite control centers...*Feed me*! Then when the busyness of the day subsides, you have a ravenous appetite. Eating throughout the day may keep the appetite control centers in check.

2. Remember when I mentioned that the body doesn't store very much carbohydrate? The liver's supply of glucose is what maintains your blood sugar level. If you don't eat carbohydrate throughout the day (the complex kinds should predominate, not simple sugars) the liver simply can't supply enough, so by the end of the day, this, combined with No. 1, adds to a powerful appetite. Unfortunately, what often happens is the tendency to devour foods high in fats and simple sugars, because they're quick and easy to prepare. And who wants to take the time to cook when you're starving?

3. Some very interesting new research is also suggesting that foods high in complex carbohydrates (veggies, grains, fruits) should predominate at breakfast (break-the-fast). Foods higher in protein, along with carbohydrates, should be eaten toward the middle of the day. This has to do with the varying effects that carbohydrates and proteins have on some of the chemicals the body produces which allow nerve cells to communicate with each other.

4. Keep in mind that stressful situations (and they happen all day long, don't they?) cause the body to use more glucose. Snacking on high-carbohydrate foods (veggies, fruits, crackers, bagels, etc.) helps keep your blood sugar level from dropping, which may lead to a craving for sweets.

All of the above work together to tell me that eating throughout the day is certainly a good idea.

Keeping Your Record

While trying to make yourself eat a specific number of calories each day probably won't work in the long run, I strongly recommend that you keep a record of what you eat. It doesn't have to be detailed to the gram. It's just the best way to see what you're really consuming on a daily basis.

You won't have to keep this record for the rest of your life. It is ideal to keep a record for up to six months, the same amount of time that you need to make yourself stick with your activity program so that it becomes a habit. You can also change your dietary habits in about that same time frame.

Just jot down what you eat right after a meal or snack. Put a little spiral notebook in your purse or pocket. Then look over your eating record every three days or so. Are you eating enough fruits and vegetables? How about grains? Enough low-fat dairy foods? Too many foods high in protein and fat? How about sweets, treats and oils? A food record is the best way to know. Before long, you'll be thinking about what you're putting into your mouth *before* you put it in, not after.

There's a sample of the record Maggie's using in the next chapter. You can use it, or make up one that works for you.

By the way, researchers are confident that if you become more active, you'll probably start eating a healthier diet as well. It's amazing how it all works together!

One Last Time: Don't Diet

With all you've probably been through over the years regarding your weight management efforts, I hope you know that "dieting" isn't the answer. You may have experienced the "yo-yo" effect—losing, gaining, and so on. While there's controversy regarding the long-term effects of the yo-yo process, there's no doubt that dieting, especially low calorie dieting, simply doesn't work.

Foreyt and Goodrick, in *Living Without Dieting*, give perhaps the best analogy I've heard with regard to low calorie diets. They say that it's like trying to hold your breath. Of course, you can hold your breath for awhile. But sooner or later, you're going to have to take another breath.

Likewise, you can force yourself to eat too few calories for awhile. But sooner or later, usually sooner, you're going to have to eat. Dieting is like holding your breath. Your body needs calories and nutrients. If you don't eat enough, it won't be long until you're "gasping for food."

Don't Give Up—It's Gradual

The consequences of repeated weight loss and regain are uncertain. Some scientists feel that it might lead to a lower metabolism, loss of muscle and an increase in percent body fat. Others disagree.

The bottom line seems to be that it's important to keep trying to get to a healthy body weight and maintain it. What makes a difference is how you go about it, and how realistic your expectations are.

Think of all the variable factors we've discussed: body size and shape, food preferences, activity preferences, responses to weight loss programs, propensity for various kinds of behavior changes. These have been attributed by various experts and organizations to a variety of areas, including genetics, early learning experiences, psychological factors, even spiritual factors!

With so many elements at work and interrelating, it is simply not realistic or possible to make a blanket recommendation that does not take individual differences into account (although certainly this is exactly what has been done by many programs for years).

For people who have bounced back and forth on the scales, achieving a stable weight over a period of time may be a success in itself. This need not be as far as it goes, but it should be recognized as a key accomplishment. Stabilizing at a higher-than-desired weight may allow some individuals to establish new attitudes or patterns of behavior that ultimately can lead to weight loss, if desired.

Don't Throw in the Towel!

Behavior change appears to take place not so much in dramatic overnight transformations as in step-by-step gradual movement toward a goal. Experts who feel that we change in stages have shown that people who achieve success often "cycle" through these stages a number of times before making the changes permanent. Being in a stage of "readiness" to change also appears to be an important factor in our ultimate results.

So it is important that we do not throw in the towel on weight management efforts when we may simply be "cycling" through the stages that will ultimately lead to the change we desire.

Some experts believe that what is critical to achieving success with the behavior change process is the quality and quantity of personal growth we are pursuing. We do not want to continue desperately grasping diet after diet and piling up failure after failure (in addition to pounds) without establishing a new foundation for succeeding at real and permanent change.

This "foundation" can be many of the things we have already discussed: self-acceptance, self-esteem or self-empowerment efforts, stress management and relaxation, spiritual practices, attention to eating disorder issues, therapy for psychological issues, pursuing information for improving coping skills in relationships, parenting, finances, work, career or creativity issues.

These efforts will not magically result in a healthy weight, but they may very well improve your ability to meet the demanding challenge of behavior change. Making some healthy choices in these areas may help you improve the choices you're making in *all* areas of your life.

Eating disorders specialist Becky Jackson says that "Healthy eating can look very much like a diet from the outside. What makes the difference is what's in your *heart*—whether you're making those choices to nourish yourself out of love, or to control yourself out of desperation and fear."

Whew! You're probably thinking, *"this doesn't sound like a very quick solution!"* That's exactly right. If changing our activity and eating habits were simple matters, statistics wouldn't indicate that at this time at least 80% of people are unable to maintain weight loss or maintain a regular habit of physical activity.

Just by reading this book and considering undertaking the complex challenge of behavior change, you have put yourself in a unique group of people who are attempting to do what a majority of people have so far not accomplished.

Congratulations! *Just remember to take your time!*

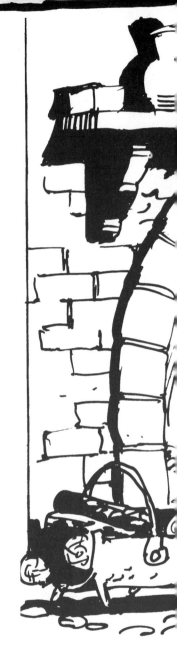

Section V. Real-Life Living
(Or, Cinderella Doesn't Live Here Anymore)

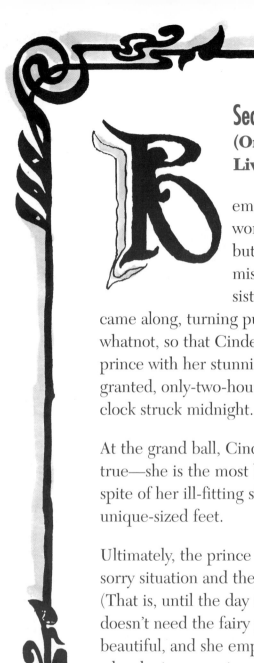

Remember Cinderella, who worked so hard to be so good, but was still ridiculed and mistreated by her evil stepsisters? A fairy godmother came along, turning pumpkins into coaches and whatnot, so that Cinderella could bedazzle the prince with her stunning fairy-godmother-granted, only-two-hours-left beauty before the clock struck midnight.

At the grand ball, Cinderella's dreams come true—she is the most beautiful of them all—in spite of her ill-fitting shoes and extraordinarily unique-sized feet.

Ultimately, the prince takes Cinderella out of her sorry situation and they live happily ever after. (That is, until the day Cinderella realizes she doesn't need the fairy godmother to make her beautiful, and she empowers herself to accept who she is, get active, eat sensibly and live healthily ever after…But that's another story! Come to think of it, that's *this* story!)

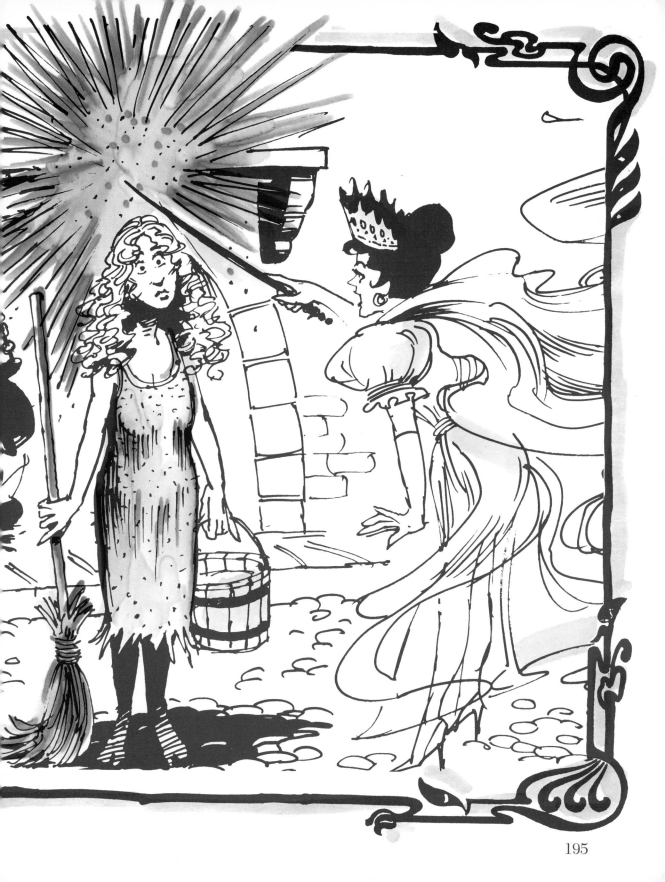

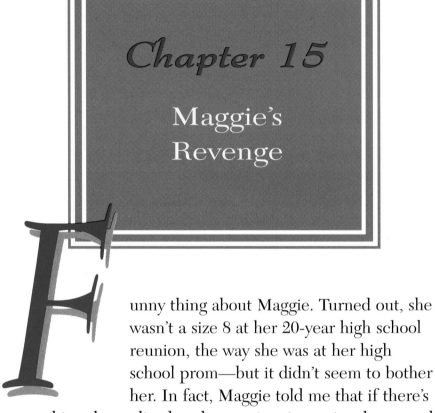

Chapter 15

Maggie's Revenge

Funny thing about Maggie. Turned out, she wasn't a size 8 at her 20-year high school reunion, the way she was at her high school prom—but it didn't seem to bother her. In fact, Maggie told me that if there's one thing she realized at the reunion, it was just how much she'd changed since the old days when all she could think about was her size.

"You know, there I was in that same high school gymnasium where I was once so miserable, and all the memories of how awful I used to feel about myself came flooding back to me," Maggie told me. "But the good thing was, it just made be realize how far I'd come! It wasn't my dress size I was thinking about when I got ready for the reunion—it was how much I liked the person I saw in the mirror and how excited I was to share 'the real me' with my old high school friends!

"I couldn't wait to tell them about my yoga class, and the step class, and the hikes Jim and I are planning for next summer. And I wanted to tell my old friends from art class that I finally got a part-time job at an ad agency, doing some graphic design.

"And I guess it didn't hurt that I had lost 14 pounds in the last six months—and I had this really great dress!"

Maggie also shared that not everyone at the reunion had tried the same technique. "At the table for awhile a group of people were talking and laughing about how they crash dieted to make a better impression at the reunion. It felt so weird not to be one of them—me, the professional dieter!

"When one of my best friends shared with me how terrible she felt about her weight, I was able to tell her that we could talk later if she wanted to know more about getting healthier, but what mattered to me most was her *friendship*, not her size. And I meant it! Not just for her, but for me, too. My friendship with me means more than my size— that's the reason I'm doing everything I can, not only to be healthy—but to be *happy*, at least as much as possible. You know, for the first time in my life, I feel like the direction toward healthier instead of heavier just might *last*! Now that would be magic.

"Don't get me wrong—you and I both know that I haven't solved all my problems or figured out how to have a perfect life, but I sure am a lot happier these days about the way I'm living."

She winked at me, and added, "I guess you could say I got real, huh?"

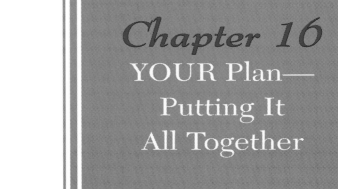

Chapter 16
YOUR Plan—
Putting It
All Together

After Maggie had a complete physical, we began to put her lifestyle plan together. Planning ahead is an important part of this process. Of course you need to be flexible, and adapt your plan as you need to. But the planning is just like charting a course. I hope the pilots who fly the planes I travel in plan their course before we leave!

The other equally important aspect is keeping records of how well the plan is going. Record keeping doesn't have to be detailed and overly time-consuming. But it really helps most of us stay on track, especially at the beginning of a new process, like lifestyle changes. It also is a great way to look back a month or two down the road to see where you are now.

As time goes by, the need for record keeping usually diminishes or disappears, since the hoped-for changes turn into new habits. But the process is always there if you need a little refresher!

At the end of this chapter, I have included eight fill-in pages that will make up your *Get Real* healthy living and weight management plan. Make copies and get started! You may not want to use all of the charts, but pick the ones that will apply best to your needs. Remember, the more you participate, the better your chances of longterm success!

Before you begin to develop the plans for yourself, let's talk briefly about how I used each of them with Maggie. Then make copies and get started.

Self-Acceptance

First, I asked Maggie to write down a daily list of at least five things that she did that day that made her feel good about herself. It could be the same things from day to day. I just wanted her to start practicing the art of accepting herself for the really good person that she is.

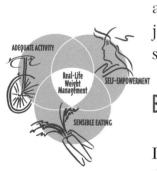

Body Image

I also asked Maggie to track her feelings about her body throughout the first six months of the program—not every day, but whenever she felt the issue was coming up for her.

Stress Management Plan

Maggie developed a list of stressful situations in her life, and a variety of strategies for handling them when they came up. We referred to this list throughout the six months.

Weekly Activity Plan

Maggie also planned, with specific days and times, when she was going to do her aerobics, cycling, walking, strength routine and stretching routine.

Since the stretching routine in Chapter 11 only takes about 10-15 minutes, Maggie has a goal of stretching 5 days a week. To get the most benefit, she stretches right after either her aerobic activity or the strength program in Chapter 10.

And she always takes at least one day off to rest. That's a very important day!

Daily and Weekly Sensible Eating

Maggie's sensible eating plan focused on servings from each group in the Food Guide Pyramid, without specifically counting calories. Here are the forms she used to create a weekly plan, and the ones she used to keep track of her daily eating habits. (The Resources section includes some references which give a detailed analysis of a multitude of foods, including calories per serving.)

Perceived Barriers and Strategies

Finally, Maggie wrote down a list of all her best "excuses" and rationalizations for not wanting to exercise or make healthy food choices, and we brainstormed for possible solutions. Not all of these worked all the time! That's just about being human. But the fact that Maggie had anticipated these situations and thought about how to counteract them left her better prepared to face them as they came up.

Get Real Healthy Lifestyle Contract With Myself

I also had Maggie sign a contract with herself to commit to becoming more active and healthy. This contract is an important part of your plan.

Support System

Maggie and I talked about various ways that she could integrate a support system into her process of change. This support network can include anyone from family and friends to formal groups to professionals including doctors, nutritionists, psychologists and fitness professionals.

At various times, Maggie relied more heavily on some methods of support than others. The important thing is that she knew the network was there when she needed it—and also that it gave her the opportunity to serve as support for others, which reinforced her feelings of self-esteem and connection to others.

Time For You To Get Started

Are you ready? It's time to put YOUR plan together. Read and copy the blank charts which follow (use Maggie's for reference).

Make copies so that you'll have enough as you work through your program for six months. Leave the ones in the book blank so that you can make more copies as you need them.

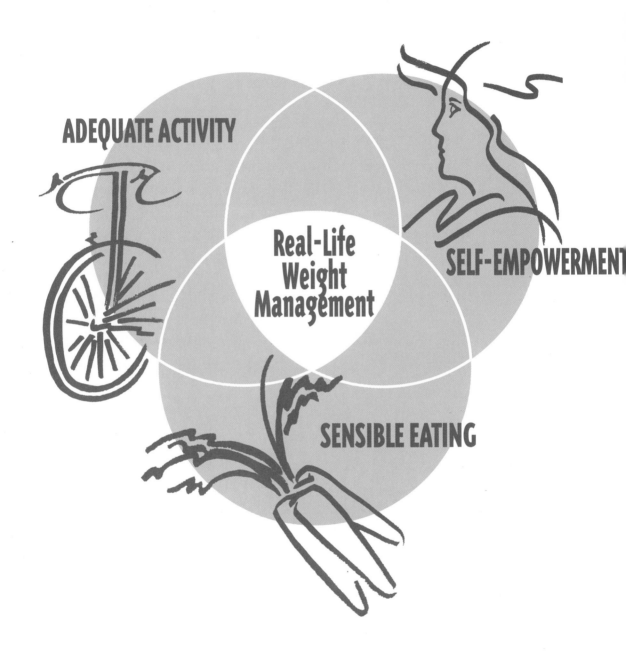

ADEQUATE ACTIVITY

SELF-EMPOWERMENT

Real-Life
Weight
Management

SENSIBLE EATING

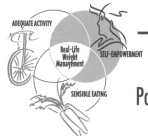

Day: _____

Five things I did today that made me feel good about myself:

1. _____

2. _____

3. _____

4. _____

5. _____

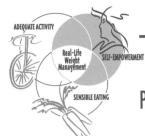

Get Real Plan

Part Two — Changing My Image of My Body

Day: _____

As you're going through the process of adopting a healthier lifestyle, it's very helpful to reflect on how you move toward a higher level of self-acceptance with body image. As often as you feel like it, hopefully at least once a week, take a moment to explore how you feel about the way you look to yourself (compared with how you felt when you first got started). Write down some thoughts that relate to these two "old beliefs."

"I will be able to love myself when I'm a size ___."

_____

"My body is not as beautiful as other people's bodies."

_____

My image of myself is changing in these ways...

_____

_____

_____

_____

_____

_____

_____

Note: This form, especially, can be tailored to your individual needs.
If you have a special body image concern, include it in your writing.

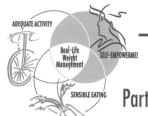

Get Real Plan

Part Three — Using Stressful Situations as a Challenge

Day: _____

Write about three stressful situations you encountered today. How did you respond? As you reflect on them, what might you try to do differently when confronted with a similar situation in the future?

1. Situation: _____

Response: _____

Future Response: _____

2. Situation: _____

Response: _____

Future Response: _____

3. Situation: _____

Response: _____

Future Response: _____

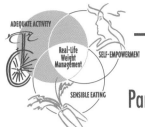

Get Real Plan

Part Four — Weekly Exercise Plan (Maggie's Sample)

Week of: _____

This is an example of Maggie's current weekly exercise plan.

Monday	Tuesday	Wednesday	Thursday	Friday	Saturday	Sunday
walking 30 minutes stretch	strength stretch	group exercise 60 minutes stretch	strength stretch	rest	cycling 50 minutes stretch	Yoga
NOTES ABOUT TODAY'S ACTIVITY						
right foot a little sore			still working on full push-ups		Rode with Jim and kids. Lots of fun.	

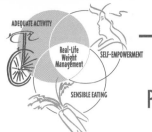

ADEQUATE ACTIVITY

Real-Life
Weight
Management

SELF-EMPOWERMENT

SENSIBLE EATING

Get Real Plan

Part Four — Weekly Exercise Plan

Week of: _____

You can develop your exercise plan in the following grid. Then, like Maggie, there's room to check off that you've stayed with your goal and make any notes you want to. Be sure to record how long your cardiovascular workouts last.

Monday	Tuesday	Wednesday	Thursday	Friday	Saturday	Sunday
NOTES ABOUT TODAY'S ACTIVITY						

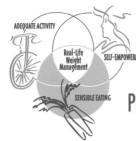

Get Real Plan

Part Five — Weekly Eating Plan (Maggie's Sample)

Week of: _____

	Monday	Tuesday	Wednesday	Thursday	Friday	Saturday	Sunday
BREAKFAST							
	1 toast (jelly) 1 banana 1 cup cereal 1 cup 1% milk coffee	2 egg omelet w/veggies 1 cup o.j. coffee	1 toast (jelly) 1/2 cup straw-berries 1 cup cereal 1 cup 1% milk coffee	1 banana 1 cup cereal 1 cup 1% milk coffee	1 orange 1 cup cereal 1 cup 1% milk 1 toast (jelly) coffee	fruit salad 2 oz. cheese coffee	3 pancakes w/syrup 1 cup 1% milk 1 tsp. tub margarine coffee
LUNCH							
	turkey breast sandwich 2 bread 1 carrot 1 cup 1% milk	tuna sandwich 2 bread 1 carrot diet soda	carrots celery pickle chicken breast sandwich 2 bread 1 cup 1% milk	large veggie salad 1 tbsp. dressing 1 cup 1% milk 2 bread	1 cheese-burger 1 fries 1 carrot celery diet soda	chicken breast sandwich 2 bread carrot sticks celery	1 cup pasta w/tomato sauce large salad 1 tbsp. dressing 1 bread diet soda
DINNER							
	4 veggie salad 1 cup pasta 1 cup 1% milk 1 cup frozen yogurt water	2 cups stew w/ lean meat, carrots, potatoes, turnips, onions 1 cup 1% milk water	1 cup cooked rice & beans 1 chicken breast (baked, no skin) 1 cup 1% milk water	3 shrimp 5 oz. lean steak salad 1 baked potato 5 straw-berries water	bean burrito w/ 2 oz. cheese & onions steamed broccoli & cauliflower 1 cup 1% milk water	vegetable lasagna large salad 1 bread water	beef stirfry steamed rice straw-berries & 1 cup low-fat yogurt water
SNACKS							
	grapes	rice cake apple	candy bar 1 cup apple juice	pretzels	2 oz. tortilla chips	1 apple popcorn (air popped)	1/3 cup almonds

AND DON'T FORGET PLENTY OF WATER, 6-8 GLASSES A DAY!

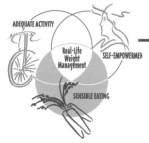

ADEQUATE ACTIVITY
Real-Life Weight Management
SELF-EMPOWERMENT
SENSIBLE EATING

Get Real Plan
Part Five — Weekly Eating Plan

Week of: _____

Monday	Tuesday	Wednesday	Thursday	Friday	Saturday	Sunday
BREAKFAST						
LUNCH						
DINNER						
SNACKS						

AND DON'T FORGET PLENTY OF WATER, 6-8 GLASSES A DAY!

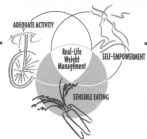

ADEQUATE ACTIVITY
Real-Life Weight Management
SELF-EMPOWERMENT
SENSIBLE EATING

Get Real Plan

Part Six — Daily Eating Record (Maggie's Sample)

Day: _____

Write down what you eat during the day. Then fill in the circles on the pyramid for the servings you eat from each group.

Breakfast ●

1 toast (1 tsp. margarine)

1 banana

1 cup cereal

coffee

1 cup 1% milk

Lunch ●

6 oz. turkey breast sandwich (mayo)

lettuce, onion, tomato

2 bread

carrot

1 cup 1% milk

Dinner ●

4 veggie salad (1 tbsp. dressing)

1 cup pasta (tomato sauce)

1 cup 1% milk

1 cup frozen yogurt

Snacks ●

1 cup grapes

3 rice cakes

Water

2 morning

2 afternoon

2 evening

1 bedtime

Fats, oils, sweets

Milk, yogurt, cheese

Meat, poultry, fish, legumes, eggs, nuts

Vegetables

Fruits

Bread, cereal, pasta, rice

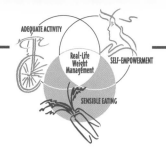

Get Real Plan

Part Six — Daily Eating Record

Day: _____

Write down what you eat during the day. Then fill in the circles on the pyramid for the servings you eat from each group.

Breakfast ◯

_____

_____

_____

Lunch ◯

_____

_____

_____

Dinner ◯

_____

_____

_____

_____

_____

Fats, oils, sweets

Milk, yogurt, cheese

Meat, poultry, fish, legumes, eggs, nuts

Vegetables

Fruits

Bread, cereal, pasta, rice

Snacks ◯

_____

_____

_____

_____

_____

Water

_____

_____

_____

_____

_____

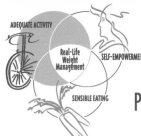

Get Real Plan

Part Seven — Overcoming Barriers to Exercise

In Chapter 8 we looked at many of the common barriers to starting or staying with regular exercise as part of your lifestyle. The best intentions can still be sidetracked by real-life issues which make it easy to begin skipping the exercise plan you've developed. Write about any barriers you experienced today which made you skip, or think about skipping, your planned activity. What did you do about it? If it made you skip today's plan, how might you handle the situation in the future so you could overcome the barrier?

Barrier: _____

Response: _____

Possible future response: _____

Barrier: _____

Response: _____

Possible future response: _____

Barrier: _____

Response: _____

Possible future response: _____

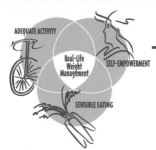

Get Real Plan

Part Eight — Contract With Myself

This is my contract with myself to live an active, healthy lifestyle. By signing this contract, I am making a commitment to live an active, healthy lifestyle on a day-by-day basis. I agree that I will:

1. Like myself for who I am right now;

2. No longer allow myself to feel that I must look like what the advertising media constantly portrays as necessary to be attractive and happy;

3. Include regular physical activity as part of my healthy lifestyle because I realize that's the best way to maintain a healthy weight;

4. Plan a weekly schedule of activities which includes aerobic, strengthening and stretching exercises;

5. Eat a sensible diet which provides plenty of whole grains, fruits, vegetables and legumes, and modest amounts of low-fat dairy and lean meat (if I choose to include meats);

6. Regularly eat breakfast, lunch and wholesome snacks throughout the day so I won't be lacking in calories which may encourage me to binge later;

7. Allow myself to occasionally enjoy the "fun foods" in my life, which I know are high in fat, without feeling guilty or like a "diet failure;"

8. Consider my eating habits as a lifestyle process, not as a short-term attempt to achieve unrealistic weight loss goals:

9. Keep records of my exercise and eating plans for up to six months from today, recognizing that after that period of time, the exercise and eating plans I develop will have become lifestyle habits; and,

10. Remember that I, like everyone, will have "good days" and "bad days" in sticking with my healthy lifestyle. The key is to not let the bad days sidetrack me. I will live my healthy lifestyle one day at a time.

_____

My name   Date   Someone who really
                                                   cares about me!

Not the End, Just a Beginning

We have reached the end of this book, but not by any means, the end of your lifestyle change process. I hope that this has been a beginning for you—an opportunity to gain some new perspectives and learn new ideas for how you can make your life as healthy and happy as possible. I hope you feel encouraged to seek out new and valuable information whenever and wherever possible.

Remember that when you use the plans outlined here, they are yours and yours alone. You're not trying to fit yourself into someone else's design. *You're learning that the best design is the one you make yourself.* That's the best way to get healthier, and reach a healthier body weight as a result of nurturing yourself on a day by day basis.

You *know* you'll face challenges and distractions. But you've got a plan for recognizing and getting past them. One key, as you know, is to plan small changes, just a little bit at a time. Be patient. Be persistent. When you get frustrated, take it as a signal that you need to be nicer to yourself—go to a movie, go to the woods, read a fairy tale. In real life, we *can* live happily ever after—especially if we take it one healthy step at a time.

Resources

Fitness Assistance
For how to find (and what to look for in) a personal trainer, fitness
instructor and/or fitness center/health club, contact:
IDEA, the international association of fitness professionals
6190 Cornerstone Court East, Suite 204
San Diego, California 92121
619-535-8979, 619-535-8234 (fax), 800-999-4332

Books

ACSM Fitness Book
1992, American College of
Sports Medicine,
Indianapolis, IN

**Binge Eating: Nature,
Assessment and Treatment**
1993, Christopher G. Fairburn
and G. Terence Wilson.
Guilford Press, 72 Spring St.
New York, NY 10012

**Bye Bye Baby Fat, Reshaping
the NEW Mother...Mind and
Body**
1994, Sandra Trexler, EdD
and Michael Trexler, PhD,
The Summit Group,
Fort Worth, TX 76104

Dieting: A Dry Drunk
1991, Becky Lu Jackson,
Nautilus Publishing
1380 Garnet Avenue
Suite #E336
San Diego, CA 92109

Fat Is a Feminist Issue
Susie Orbach,
Berkley Publishers

**Fat is not a Four-
Letter Word.**
1992, Charles Roy Schroeder,
PhD, CHRONIMED
Publishing, PO Box 47945,
Minneapolis, MN 55447

The Feeling Good Handbook
1989, David Burns, MD,
Penguin Group
375 Hudson Street
New York, NY 10014

First Things First
1994, Stephen R. Covey, A.
Roger Merrill, and Rebecca R.
Merrill, Simon and Schuster,
Rockefeller Center,
123 Avenue of the Americas,
New York, NY 10020

**Food Values of Portions
Commonly Used, 14th ed.**
1985, Jean Pennington, PhD,
RD and Helen Church,
Harper and Row,
New York, NY

Healthy Pleasures
1989, Robert Ornstein, PhD
and David Sobel, MD,
Addison-Wesley Publishing
Co., Inc.

**Jane Brody's
Nutrition Book**
Bantam Books, 1985,
W. W. Norton, 500 5th Ave.,
New York, NY 10110

**The LEARN Program for
Weight Control**
1989, Kelly D. Brownell, PhD,
American Health
Publishing Co.
(800) 736-7323

Living with Exercise
Stephen Blair, PED,
American Health Publishing,
Dallas, TX
(800) 736-7323

Living Without Dieting
1994, John P. Foreyt, PhD,
and G. Ken Goodrick, PhD,
1992, Warner Books, Harrison
Publishing, Houston, TX
(800) 945-6199

**Love the Body You Were
Born With**
1994, Monica Dixon, MS, RD,
San Francisco, CA
(800) 936-7978

Nutrition Desk Reference
1985, Robert Garrison, Jr.,
MA, RPh, Elizabeth Somer,
MA, RD, Keats Publishing,
New Canaan, CT

Nutrition for Women
1993, Elizabeth Somer, MA,
RD, Henry Holt and
Company, 115 W. 118th Street,
New York, NY 10011

Perfect Weight
1991, Deepak Chopra, MD,
Harmony Books,
Crown Publishers,
201 East 50th Street,
New York, NY 10022

Physiology of Fitness
3rd ed.
1990, Brian Sharkey, PhD,
Human Kinetics Publishers,
PO Box 5076, Champaign, IL
61825 (800) 747-4457

A Woman's Book of Strength
Training
1995, Karen Andes, Perigee
Books/Berkley Publishers

Your Maximum Mind
Herbert Benson, Avon Books,
105 Madison Ave.,
New York, NY 10016

Books with Recipes

Butter Busters: The Cookbook
Butter Busters Publishing, Inc.
PO Box 150562
Arlingon, TX 76015
(817) 478-9359

Fat Free Living,
Vol. 1 and 2
Jyl Steinback, Fat Free Living,
Inc., Scottsdale, AZ
(602) 996-6300

In the Kitchen
With Rosie
1994, Rosie Daley, Random
House Publishers

Jane Brody's Good
Food Book
1985, Bantam Books, W. W.
Norton, 500 5th Ave., New
York, NY 10110

Meal Planning and
Recipe Products

The Think Lite Program
Speaking of Fitness
SOF, Inc.
The Lowfat Living Co.
98 Everett Drive, Suite C,
Durango, CO 81301
(303) 247-3610

Support Groups

Overeater's Anonymous
PO Box 92870
Los Angeles, CA 90009
(213) 936-6252

Magazines/Newsletters

SHAPE
451 Park Ave. S.
New York, NY 10016

New Woman
215 Lexingon Ave.
New York, NY 10016

Cooking Light: The Magazine
of Food and Fitness
PO Box 830549
Birmington, AL 35282
(800) 999-1750

Nutrition Action Newsletter
Center for Science in the
Public Interest
1875 Connecticut Ave. NW,
Suite 300
Washington, DC 20009
(202) 667-7483

Eating Disorders Information

International Association of
Eating Disorders Professionals
123 NW 13th Street
Suite 206
Boca Raton, FL 33432
(407) 338-6494 (for referral to
a therapist in your area)

Becky L. Jackson
Recovery Center
B.L. Jackson & Associates
1380 Garnet Avenue
Suite E-336,
San Diego, CA 92109
(619) 278-8050

Catalogues/Products

Calorie Control Council
5775 Peachtree-Dunwoody
Road, Suite 500-G
Atlanta, GA 30342
(404) 252-3663

Creative Health
Products Catalogue
(heart rate monitors,
exercise equipment, etc.)
5148 Saddle Ridge Road
Plymouth, MI 48105
(800) 742-4478

Lowfat Lifeline
52 Condolea Court
Lake Oswego, OR 97035
(503) 636-1559

Nutritionist IV
(software for food/diet analysis)
N-Squared Computing
First Databank Division
The Hearst Corporation
1111 Bayhill Dr., Suite 350
San Bruno, CA 94066
(415) 266-8016,
(800) 289-1701

Audios/Videos

Jane Fonda's Yoga
Exercise Workout
(videotape)
Jane Fonda's Lean Routine
(videotape)
(800) 824-7148

Kathy Smith's "New Yoga"
Workout
(videotape)
Kathy Smith's "Walk-Fit" Tape
(audio tape)
BodyVision
75 Rockefeller Plaza
New York, NY 10019
(212) 275-2900
(800) 95-WARNER

Kari Anderson's
Tone It Up! (videotape)
Pro-Robics Video, Inc.
1530 Queen Anne Ave. N.
Seattle, WA 98109
(800) 537-5512

About the Author

Daniel Kosich, PhD, who received his doctorate from Brigham Young University, has been helping professionals and consumers apply the science of health and fitness for the past 15 years. He is currently a Senior Consultant for IDEA in San Diego, and the president of EXERFIT Lifestyle Consulting in Denver.

He is also co-exercise science editor for *SHAPE* magazine, and a contributing editor for *New Woman* magazine. As the former program director for the Jane Fonda Workout and currently their technical consultant, Dr. Kosich has contributed to over 15 Jane Fonda fitness video programs, including development of the script for the weight control segment of the "Jane Fonda Lean Routine" video. He is an internationally respected speaker and author of numerous magazine articles on fitness and health.

Starting Your Own GET REAL Healthy Living Group

GET REAL Healthy Living Groups focus on the positive aspects of learning from others by sharing ways to apply the concepts described in *GET REAL*.

As part of your *GET REAL* group, you'll have the opportunity to find an exercise partner or someone to share recipes and restaurants with. And you're *sure* to find support in feeling good about yourself every day!

If you're interested in finding out how to start your own *GET REAL* Healthy Living Group, please send the coupon below along with $1.00 and a self-addressed, stamped envelope to:

GET REAL Healthy Living Group
IDEA
6190 Cornerstone Ct. East, Suite 204
San Diego, CA 92121-3773

Want the latest information on health and fitness or additional copies of *GET REAL*?

Fill out the coupon below or call (800) 999-4332, ext. 7, or (619) 535-8979, Mon.-Fri., 9:00 AM-5:00 PM Pacific time.

- - - - - - - - - - - ✂ -

Check one

❑ Please send me information on starting a *GET REAL* Healthy Living Group. I have enclosed $1.00 and a self-addressed, stamped envelope.

❑ Please add me to your mailing list so I can continue to receive the latest health and fitness information.

❑ I'd like to order additional copies of *GET REAL: A Personal Guide To Real-Life Weight Management*. I have enclosed $15.95 plus $2.50 for shipping and handling for each copy (CA residents, add 7% sales tax). Product number C895016.

Name _____

Address _____

City _____ State/Province _____

County _____ Zip/Postal Code _____